The Medical Library Association Guide to Developing Consumer Health Collections

MEDICAL LIBRARY ASSOCIATION BOOKS

The Medical Library Association (MLA) features books that showcase the expertise of health sciences librarians for other librarians and professionals.

MLA Books are excellent resources for librarians in hospitals, medical research practice, and other settings. These volumes will provide health care professionals and patients with accurate information that can improve outcomes and save lives.

Each book in the series has been overseen editorially since conception by the Medical Library Association Books Panel, composed of MLA members with expertise spanning the breadth of health sciences librarianship.

Medical Library Association Books Panel

Kristen L. Young, AHIP, chair
Dorothy Ogdon, AHIP, chair designate
Michel C. Atlas
Carolann Lee Curry
Kelsey Leonard, AHIP
Karen McElfresh, AHIP
JoLinda L. Thompson, AHIP
Heidi Heilemann, AHIP, board liaison

About the Medical Library Association

Founded in 1898, MLA is a 501(c)(3) nonprofit, educational organization of 3,500 individual and institutional members in the health sciences information field that provides lifelong educational opportunities, supports a knowledge base of health information research, and works with a global network of partners to promote the importance of quality information for improved health to the health care community and the public.

Books in the Series:

The Medical Library Association Guide to Providing Consumer and Patient Health Information edited by Michele Spatz
Health Sciences Librarianship edited by M. Sandra Wood
Curriculum-Based Library Instruction: From Cultivating Faculty Relationships to Assessment edited by Amy Blevins and Megan Inman
The Small Library Manager's Handbook by Alice Graves
Mobile Technologies for Every Library by Ann Whitney Gleason

The Medical Library Association Guide to Answering Questions about the Affordable Care Act edited by Emily Vardell

Marketing for Special and Academic Libraries: A Planning and Best Practices Sourcebook by Patricia Higginbottom and Valerie Gordon

Interprofessional Education and Medical Libraries: Partnering for Success edited by Mary E. Edwards

Translating Expertise: The Librarian's Role in Translational Research edited by Marisa L. Conte

Expert Searching in the Google Age by Terry Ann Jankowski

Digital Rights Management: The Librarian's Guide edited by Catherine A. Lemmer and Carla P. Wale

The Medical Library Association Guide to Data Management for Librarians edited by Lisa Federer

Developing Librarian Competencies for the Digital Age edited by Jeffrey Coghill and Roger Russell

New Methods of Teaching and Learning in Libraries by Ann Whitney Gleason

Becoming a Powerhouse Librarian: How to Get Things Done Right the First Time by Jamie Gray

Assembling the Pieces of a Systematic Review: A Guide for Librarians edited by Margaret J. Foster and Sarah T. Jewell

Information and Innovation: A Natural Combination for Health Sciences Libraries edited by Jean P. Shipman and Barbara A. Ulmer

The Library Staff Development Handbook: How to Maximize Your Library's Most Important Resource by Mary Grace Flaherty

Transforming Medical Library Staff for the Twenty-First Century edited by Melanie J. Norton and Nathan Rupp

Health Sciences Collection Management for the Twenty-First Century edited by Susan K. Kendall

The Medical Library Association Guide to Developing Consumer Health Collections by Claire B. Joseph

The Medical Library Association Guide to Developing Consumer Health Collections

Claire B. Joseph

ROWMAN & LITTLEFIELD
Lanham • Boulder • New York • London

Published by Rowman & Littlefield
A wholly owned subsidiary of The Rowman & Littlefield Publishing Group, Inc.
4501 Forbes Boulevard, Suite 200, Lanham, Maryland 20706
www.rowman.com

Unit A, Whitacre Mews, 26-34 Stannary Street, London SE11 4AB

Copyright © 2018 by Medical Library Association

All rights reserved. No part of this book may be reproduced in any form or by any electronic or mechanical means, including information storage and retrieval systems, without written permission from the publisher, except by a reviewer who may quote passages in a review.

British Library Cataloguing in Publication Information Available

Library of Congress Cataloging-in-Publication Data Available

ISBN 9781442281691 (hardback : alk. paper) | ISBN 9781442281707 (pbk. : alk. paper) | ISBN 9781442281714 (electronic)

∞™ The paper used in this publication meets the minimum requirements of American National Standard for Information Sciences—Permanence of Paper for Printed Library Materials, ANSI/NISO Z39.48-1992.

Printed in the United States of America

To my beloved mother,
Lillian Emmerich Joseph (1920–1995)
My first and best teacher

Contents

List of Figures	xi
List of Tables	xiii
List of Sample Forms	xv
Preface	xvii
Acknowledgments	xxi
1 How and Where to Begin: The Main Ingredients	1
2 Your Library's Neighborhood and Its Effects on the Health of Your Community	15
3 Building the Collection	23
4 Grants	49
5 Staff Customer Service	57
6 Library Privacy and Confidentiality	65
7 Community Outreach Planning	83
8 Health Literacy and Librarians	97
9 Multicultural/Inclusive Consumer Health Information	109
10 Where Consumers Go to Find Health Information: Apps, Social Media, and Wikipedia	123

| 11 | Consumer Health Information Outreach for Every Library | 135 |

Index 145

About the Author 151

List of Figures

Figure 1.1.	Randy Glasbergen cartoon	2
Figure 3.1.	Mount Carmel Consumer Health Information LibGuide	25
Figure 3.2.	MedlinePlus screen shot	28
Figure 3.3.	Mount Carmel Consumer Health Library Collection Development & Management Policy	35
Figure 5.1.	Volunteer ready to serve	61

List of Tables

Table 1.1.	Budget Types	11
Table 7.1.	Logic Model Template	86
Table 7.2.	Logic Model Complete	87
Table 7.3.	Worksheet Blank—Process Assessment Questions & Methods	90
Table 7.4.	Worksheet Blank—Objectives & Methods	91

List of Sample Forms

Sample Form 3.1.	Preston Medical Library	37
Sample Form 6.1.	New York Public Library Privacy Policy	71
Sample Form 6.2.	The National Network of Libraries of Medicine, "The Consumer Health Reference Interview and Ethical Issues"	77
Sample Form 7.1.	Four-Step Proposal Writing (NNLM NEO)	93
Sample Form 9.1.	IFLA/UNESCO Multicultural Library Manifesto	111
Sample Form 10.1.	HealthIT.gov Guidelines: Find Quality Resources in e-Health	125

Preface

Many baby boomers remember that in their childhood, doctors made house calls along with all the decisions about their patients' health care. Sweeping societal changes over the decades included the demand for patients' rights, changing patients' role in their health care from a passive to an active one. Sweeping changes in health care and its delivery and clinician reimbursements from both private insurance companies and government programs forced clinicians to see more patients but devote less time to them. And as author Fredrik Backman so wryly observes, physicians often speak to their patients "with a series of terms that no human being with less than ten years of medical training or an entirely unhealthy addiction to certain television series could ever be expected to understand" (2012, 328). The result is that it has become increasingly difficult to navigate in today's health-care experience. In an information-rich society it's positively disheartening to learn that many are unable to understand their healthcare issues and what to do about them, especially when this ignorance remains after a patient-clinician exchange. Patients really have no choice but to become their own advocates and try to find the information they need to enable them to make educated decisions ultimately in partnership with their clinicians.

This reality has made it imperative for all libraries to devote at least a part of their collections to consumer health information—information written for nonclinicians. Librarians chose a service profession and both personally and professionally are dedicated to providing their patrons with the best information available.

How to define a consumer health library? There really is no "one size fits all" definition. As Jean Shipman and Erica Lake perceptively observe, "If you've seen one consumer health library, you have seen one consumer health library" (2014, 77). Consumer health collections can run the gamut from online LibGuides and databases, and a few shelves devoted to consumer health materials, to a freestanding library whose raison d'être is a consumer health collection. And libraries can be public;

academic; part of a medical, nursing, or allied health school; a private autonomous hospital; or one that is part of a massive health-care system.

The aim of this work is to be an information resource for all librarians, from the student or novice to the seasoned veteran, and everyone in between. It can be treated as a reference work, with each chapter devoted to a part of the whole. While primarily for the novice, with all the ingredients needed to create and maintain a consumer health library collection, there are included examples of just some of the innumerable, diverse, imaginative, creative, purposeful, and successful consumer health outreach programs and initiatives librarians have accomplished throughout the country. These will serve to inspire and encourage all librarians to create their own community outreach. The sky's the limit!

Librarians face two main challenges in connecting excellent consumer health information with their patrons. The first is society's pervasive mind-set, which cuts a wide swath across ages, ethnicities, socioeconomic status, and educational levels, that the internet makes those in search of information, including health information, self-sufficient, no longer needing an intermediary (like a librarian!) to help them find what they need. Turning to "Dr. Google" may very well yield results, but are the results accurate and from reliable sources? For the most part the consumer accepts its information unvetted, with little or no knowledge of its sources (and certainly not evaluating them). Unfortunately for many, "they don't know what they don't know." Everyone should heed the wisdom of well-known graphic novelist Neil Gaiman:

> Google can bring you back, you know, 100,000 answers. A librarian can bring you back the right one. (Gaiman 2010)

Paradoxically in this information-rich world, a significant part of the population are medically underserved and truly do not know how to access good health care, let alone where and how to find information. Ironically they are often the ones who need this information the most.

Serving this part of the community is the second major challenge librarians face. While completing the all-important needs assessment will identify these parts of the library's community, forging partnerships will play a major role in outreach programs. Community outreach is also part of the equation; community stakeholders are invaluable and must be identified, and relationships must be forged and nurtured.

With this work as a guide, every library will be able to provide quality consumer health information to its community, and the reader will find how many libraries are successfully handling this major need.

BOOK ORGANIZATION

This work can be treated as a reference work; each chapter can stand on its own.

In chapter 1, "How and Where to Begin: The Main Ingredients," readers will learn how to conduct an all-important community needs assessment, how to find and establish relationships with community stakeholders; how to write a strategic plan and a library budget, and how to approach library space planning.

Chapter 2, "Your Library's Neighborhood and Its Effects on the Health of Your Community," discusses how the different types of communities (city, rural, suburb), the natural and built environment, the climate, and other issues impact the health of the residents. Also discussed is how librarians can use this information to custom-tailor consumer information to their customers' needs.

In chapter 3, "Building the Collection," a number of sources are discussed, including online and print sources, both free and fee based. In addition, how to write a collection development and a mission statement is explained.

Chapter 4 is all about grants, how to find them, how to apply for them, and how to write a grant proposal.

Staff customer service is covered in chapter 5, including customer service training for all library employees from volunteers to professionals, along with specific training for consumer health libraries.

In chapter 6, "Library Privacy and Confidentiality," what degree of privacy and confidentiality is required by libraries is explained, and how to provide customers with the level they expect is discussed.

In chapter 7, community outreach planning is explained step by step, including how to write a logic model, measure results, and create marketing strategies.

In chapter 8, the issue of health literacy is covered, including defining what it is, how much of the population is affected by this, how it impacts their health-care knowledge and experience, and what librarians can do to help with this important issue.

Chapter 9 is devoted to finding multicultural and inclusive consumer health information, including information in multiple languages. Every library must create and maintain an inviting, nonjudgmental environment where everyone who walks through the library's door is made to feel welcome; in addition, the collection must include consumer health information for everyone.

All librarians need to be informed of just exactly where their patrons are going to find out health information, including apps, social media, and Wikipedia. Chapter 10, "Where Customers Go to Find Health Information: Apps, Social Media, and Wikipedia," explains how librarians can steer customers to the best sources of information, and how libraries can make use of social media for outreach.

Chapter 11, "Consumer Health Information Outreach for Every Library," describes programming that illustrates how libraries of any size or any budget can provide outreach services and take their library to their community.

Throughout the chapters the reader will find examples of policies, models, and forms discussed, along with some illustrations that highlight the chapters. As the author strongly believes that one of the best ways to learn is by real-life examples, just some of the innumerable innovative and creative programs librarians have successfully implemented to get the very best consumer health information to their communities are described throughout the book.

REFERENCES

Backman, Fredrik. 2012. *A Man Called Ove.* New York: Washington Square.

Gaiman, Neil. 2010. "Neil Gaiman on Libraries." YouTube video. (Excerpt starts at 1:20 of 1:56.) Video description: "Neil Gaiman, author and Honorary Chair of National Library Week, interviewed by Jon Barnes of the Indianapolis Marion County Public Library, speaks about the value of libraries, librarians and librarianship before his lecture at the annual McFadden Memorial Lecture Series hosted by Indianapolis Marion County Public Library on April 16, 2010." https://www.youtube.com/watch?v=uH-sR1uCQ6g.

Shipman, Jean, and Erica Lake. 2014. "Prized Assets: Staff." In *The Medical Library Association Guide to Providing Consumer and Patient Health Information*, edited by Michele Spatz, 77–96. Lanham, MD: Rowman & Littlefield.

Acknowledgments

I would first like to thank the Books Panel Committee of the Medical Library Association for choosing my proposal to write this book. And I must thank my editor at Rowman & Littlefield, Charles Harmon, and his most able assistant, Kathleen E. "Katie" O'Brien, for their guidance.

I would also like to extend my heartfelt thanks to my friend and colleague, Paul Moglia, PhD, Associate Program Director, South Nassau Communities Hospital Family Practice Residency Program, for his unwavering support and encouragement.

And I must give very special thanks to my fellow members of the South Nassau Communities Hospital Nursing Research/Evidence Based Practice Council, co-chaired by Marybeth Ryan, PhD, RN, Nurse Scientist, South Nassau Communities Hospital, and Jacki Rosen, MS, RN, PMHCNS-BC, Psych/Mental Health Clinical Nurse Specialist, Department of Education, South Nassau Communities Hospital. This group of nurses exemplifies all that is best in their profession. Not only are they dedicated to their work, but they are equally committed to advancing their profession through research. They are a constant source of inspiration for me.

1

How and Where to Begin

The Main Ingredients

Takeaways from this chapter:

- *The vital importance of providing library customers with accurate, up-to-date, and reliable consumer health information*
- *How to conduct a needs assessment of the library's community members*
- *How to reach out to and establish relationships with community stakeholders*
- *How to write a strategic plan for the library*
- *How to plan library space for the consumer health collection*
- *How to prepare the library's budget*

It's indisputable that all libraries need to provide reliable and authoritative consumer health information for their customers. This remains true whether the library is small, medium, or large, public, academic, or hospital or health-center based.

And this is true now more than ever. According to the Pew Research Center (2013), 72 percent of Americans say they sought health information online in the past year, and 77 percent of online health information seekers say they began with a search engine. And there are also a variety of ways to access the internet, including stationary desktops, transportable laptops, and the increasingly ubiquitous cell and smartphones. Paradoxically, the explosion of available health information does not necessarily mean that users find, or even know how to find, reliable, accurate information. There seems to be a pervasive popular mind-set, one that cuts across ages, ethnicities, socioeconomic status, and educational achievement level, that the internet, specifically a search engine like Google, is not only the best way but *the* way to find any and all information, including health information, and information sources are consulted indiscriminately with the user rarely investigating if the source of the information is accurate or reliable. This is simply because users often don't think there is any necessity to do this; quite simply put, they don't know what they don't know.

The cartoon by Randy Glasbergen in figure 1.1 wryly illustrates this pervasive mind-set.

Now this is not to suggest for a moment that the internet is a minefield of misinformation, but there is no margin of error for accurate health information, which can, at times, be quite literally a matter of life and death. But most internet users simply do not realize the importance of knowing the source of their information. This is something that librarians need to rectify, as there is such a plethora of accurate

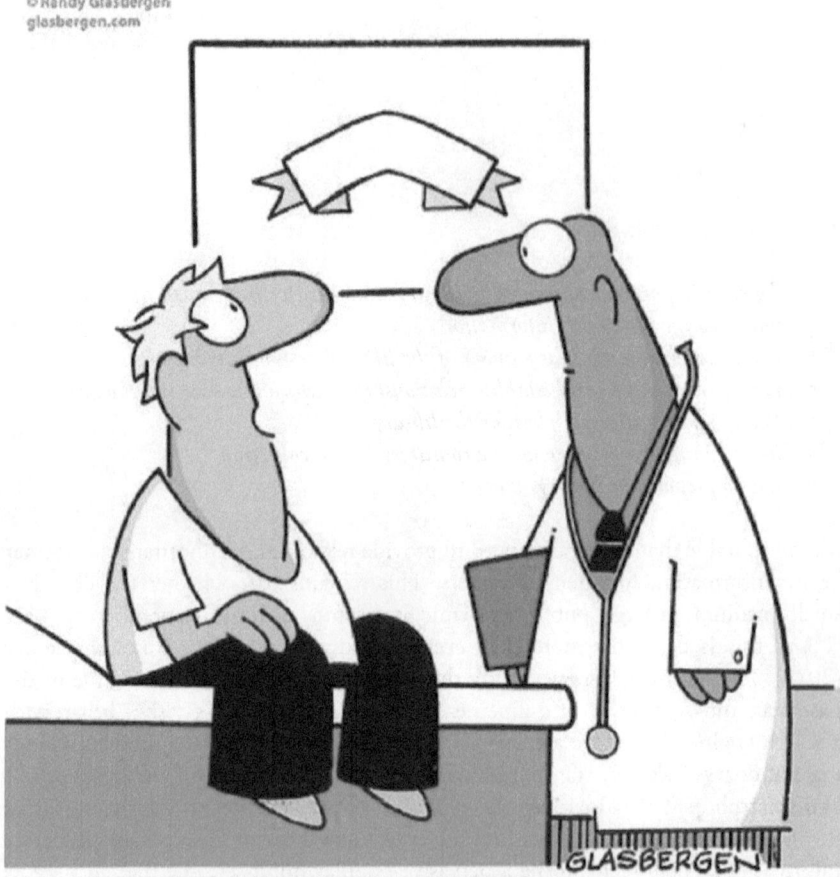

"I already diagnosed myself on the Internet. I'm only here for a second opinion."

Figure 1.1. Randy Glasbergen cartoon
Cartoon by Randy Glasbergen. Glasbergen Cartoon Service.

and reliable resources that there is no reason to use sources that "might" be correct. Adding to the necessity of providing customers with authoritative consumer health information is the climate of today's health-care system with its increasingly complex navigation and its short patient-provider interactions. Most patients are expected to be their own health advocates and learn all there is to know about their health issues, or they must rely on a relative or friend to act as their proxy.

In addition, poor health literacy is a growing problem. The Institute of Medicine's (2004) landmark report *Health Literacy: A Prescription to End Confusion* defines health literacy as "the degree to which individuals can obtain, process, and understand the basic health information and they need to make appropriate health decisions." Simply put, many patients do not understand the information their clinician is telling them, which includes how to care for themselves and medication instructions. In fact, health literacy is such a concern that the AHRQ (Agency for Healthcare Research and Quality of the US Department of Health and Human Services) created the "AHRQ Health Literacy Universal Precautions Toolkit" (updated to a 2nd edition in 2015) advising clinicians to assume that all patients may have difficulty understanding health information and utilizing services. This toolkit is available free on the internet (https://www.ahrq.gov/sites/default/files/publications/files/healthlittoolkit2_3.pdf).

And then there is the segment of society that is underprivileged and underserved, who also have insufficient or, in some cases, no equitable access to, adequate health care, let alone health information.

Suffice it to say that librarians must be proactive standard bearers for guiding their community to the best sources of health information and helping them find answers to their health questions and concerns. Consumer health collections must be part of every library of every type and size.

So where and how to begin developing a consumer health collection? Many factors are involved, including finding or making space for the collection, determining what the collection should consist of, staffing, and, of course, finding adequate funding. However, in order to provide a library's customers with the best collection and services, the first and most important step is determining exactly who those customers, the library's community, are and how their needs will be best served.

NEEDS ASSESSMENT

Whether the consumer health collection is part of a public library, a college or university library, or a hospital or academic center health sciences library, there are basic questions that must be answered and information gathered. The library needs a clear and precise portrait of its community.

Who are the library's customers? And what are the community's health issues and risks? A needs assessment would entail discovering the demographics of the community, which includes ages, socioeconomic status, educational levels, languages spoken, and ethnicities. As Dettmar points out, this places "the emphasis . . . on the development and provision of resources and services to meet library customers' identified needs based on data rather than library staff's assumption" (2014, 11–12).

Where to find this information? A number of tools will provide this, including the following:

For overall national statistics:

- US Bureau of the Census (http://www.census.gov)
- American Fact Finder (http://factfinder.census.gov)
- Easy Stats (http://www.census.gov/easystats)

For state health facts

- Community Health Status Indicators (CHSI) from the CDC
  - Health profiles for all 3,143 counties in the United States
- Community Health Needs Assessment (https://communitycommons.org/chna)
  - This tool was built to assist hospitals and organizations across the US to better understand the health needs of their community to partner for programs to improve the community's health and quality of life at local and regional levels. This was created by Community Commons, which provides access to thousands of meaningful data layers that allow the user to thoroughly explore county health. Includes video on how to use the website.
- State Health Facts from the Henry J. Kaiser Family Foundation (http://kff.org/statedata)
  - "Health Status Indicators" covers a number of topics, including "Life Expectancy," "Mental Health," "Smoking," "Cancer," "Diabetes," "Heart Disease," "Asthma," and "Obesity."
- County Health Rankings & Roadmaps (http://countyhealthrankings.org)
  - From the Robert Wood Johnson Foundation and the University of Wisconsin Population Health Institute: a source for detailed county health information
- Rural Health Information Hub (RHIhub) (https://www.ruralhealthinfo.org/topics/rural-health-research-assessment-evaluation)
  - Funded by the Federal Office of Rural Health Policy, a national clearinghouse on rural health issues. Rural communities are often underserved. Includes information on program evaluation and a link to a tool, the "Community Health Needs Assessment Toolkit" (http://ruralhealthworks.org/wp-content/files/2-CHNA-Toolkit-Text-and-All-Appendices-May-2012.pdf). The toolkit was written for hospitals, but certainly, much information can be gleaned from it. And don't overlook the importance of starting local, with the library's city or town, county, and state health department information.
  - As an example, the Department of Health, Division of Quality Improvement, Epidemiology and Research of Nassau County, New York, located on

Long Island, New York, published the *Community Health Assessment 2014–2017*. This offers an absolute wealth of demographic and health information and is openly available on the internet.

- Nassau County, with a population of over one million, is ranked as the twelfth-wealthiest county in the country and ranks eighth out of the sixty-two New York State counties in terms of health outcomes, based upon morbidity and mortality data (NCDH, n.d., 8). Yet there remain pockets of severely underserved residents, areas of low income with populations facing health risks disproportionately from other parts of Nassau. Asthma, type 2 diabetes, liver disease, and COPD rates are significantly higher in nine identified communities than in the rest of the county (NCDH, n.d., 9). These are key factors for these specific communities to address.
- Suffolk County, Long Island's easternmost county, published a similar study, *The Suffolk County Community Health Assessment 2014–2017* (SCDHS, n.d.), which, like its Nassau counterpart, also offers a wealth of information and is freely available on the internet. (Long Island geographically actually consists of four counties, but the westernmost, Queens and Kings [Brooklyn], are boroughs of Manhattan [NYC]; when people refer to Long Island they invariably mean Nassau and Suffolk.)

Does the community have a significant immigrant population? If so, information on their language, culture, and health-care customs is important. Several websites will help identify the number of immigrants in your area and their country of origin. They include:

- The Migration Policy Institute (http://www.migrationpolicy.org), an "independent, nonpartisan, nonprofit think tank in Washington, DC"; it covers demographics, language and education, workforce, and income.
- Office of Refugee Resettlement (https://www.acf.hhs.gov/orr), part of the US Department of Health and Human Services. This is primarily a wonderful resource for helping refugees, but it does also offer a look at refugees' numbers and countries of origin by state.

And don't forget: Approach local hospitals, health centers, and universities as sources of community demographics—not to mention partnerships—as they need to have this information. For example, in New York State, hospitals are required by both the state and federal governments to conduct a community health needs assessment every three years and then develop a Community Service Plan to respond to the community's health needs. These plans are available to the public and are usually found on the hospital's website, and hard copies are available. These plans will provide useful information regarding the health-care issues of the communities the hospital serves. South Nassau Communities Hospital's *Community Service Plan 2016–2018* (https://www.southnassau.org/uploads/public/documents/brochures/

csp.pdf) relates its community outreach programs on diabetes, smoking cessation, healthy food/beverage choices, cardiac disease, and stroke education. Not only does the topic of these programs give some indication of the health issues of concern to the community, but it also offers possible partnerships for the libraries in the community to provide consumer health materials. In addition, this hospital's plan lists a number of community-based organizations, with their websites; some are local branches of national organizations (e.g., the American Cancer Society), but some are homegrown, including the Asthma Coalition of Long Island and the Epilepsy Foundation of Long Island.

State health departments are also resources of disease-specific, community-specific information. For example, New York State Department of Health's Cancer Incidence by zip code offers data on four types of cancer: colorectal, female breast, lung and bronchus, and prostate.

ESTABLISHING RELATIONSHIPS WITH COMMUNITY STAKEHOLDERS

While it is absolutely imperative to have detailed demographic information for planning, these are the "cold, hard facts." Equally important is utilizing the "warm, human touch," by reaching out to community stakeholders, those with a vested interest in the health of their, for example, specific immigrant populations or ethnicities, and providing them with the best information resources. These identified stakeholders will become sounding boards for outreach programs and partners; they should be considered "vital friends" (Cuban 2007, 79). Three basic methods to gather data are:

- Interviews: Sitting down with identified and selected individuals from the community for approximately one hour
- Focus groups: The library should first decide how many focus groups there need to be, based on chosen topics, and then how many participants per group. These groups should be led by a facilitator and last for approximately ninety minutes.
- Surveys: Online surveys can be sent to identified and selected community leaders, and they can be given up to a month to return it.
  Note: Whether it's online or in print, the rate of return of surveys can be disappointingly low. However, they can yield important information.

While outreach can be accomplished by written, online, or telephone surveys, for the best outcomes, in-person interviews and focus groups are preferable, especially in the public library arena, as a public library is a readily identifiable community center. In this way, library staff is able to sit face-to-face with their customers and have conversations to find out their consumer health information needs and concerns and how they would feel best served by the library.

An excellent reference source from the National Network of Libraries of Medicine (NNLM) Pacific Northwest Region, *Measuring the Difference: Guide to Planning and Evaluating Health Information Outreach* observes:

> Depending on your community, stakeholders could include:
>
> - Health providers
> - Health care administrators
> - Continuing education officers
> - Public or rural health officials
> - Faculty
> - Consumers
> - Health educators
> - School nurses
> - State and local health personnel (Burroughs and Wood 2000, 6)

The community's houses of worship, or faith-based organizations, Boys and Girls Scouts, and other service and civic groups should also be included.

While these approaches can be used in all types of libraries, libraries that are parts of larger institutions, such as hospital libraries, have their own specific considerations. Many must go through administration and/or hospital-wide departments and committees that approve allotment of space and resources, and nonclinical, non-revenue-earning departments (like libraries) may not receive top—or even near the top—priority in these areas.

As Michelynn McKnight so pointedly observes, "Administrators are not born with a 'librarian appreciation gene'" (2011, 2), so proactive efforts by the hospital library staff to not only make their presence and services widely promoted, but to also participate in institution-wide committees including nursing education, community outreach, patient and family education, should be integral and dynamic parts of their operation. Such partnerships can also provide the library with "champions" in its quest to create consumer health collections.

Nicole Dettmar (2014, 19) spoke with Stevo Roksandic, the dynamic director of the Mount Carmel Health Sciences Library, which includes an outstanding consumer health collection, and he recounted the steps taken in their needs assessment. The result is that the library went from three hundred square feet in March 2011 to a new location with 2,400 square feet (eight times larger!) in October 2013. Some of the steps the library staff took are outlined below:

- As part of a health center, the library reached out to the nursing patient education department, which provided statistics about the diagnostic frequency of chronic diseases; this enabled the library to develop a large number of health pamphlets to meet the needs of the nursing health center.
- They reached out to nearby Kent State University School of Library and Information Science to find out their practicum assignments.

- The library staff noted that patrons preferred learning how to navigate the internet for online health information resources rather than use books, even though books could be checked out.
- The staff explored the consumer health needs of resident physicians in the hospital's clinic, which resulted in a collaborative relationship between clinicians and the consumer health library; patients were referred to the library for information regarding their health issues (along with clear disclaimers that the library staff were providing information only).
- Public librarians were consulted to find out their patrons' needs and to encourage them to refer their patrons to Mount Carmel when they needed more comprehensive information regarding their health issue.
- A partnership was established with a local assisted living community, where the facility provided space and allowed Mount Carmel consumer health library staff to promote their services there.

A needs assessment plan allows a library to have a firm understanding of its community and their consumer health information needs; it also provides hard numbers to present to administration to promote and advance the library's plans.

STRATEGIC PLAN

All libraries need to create a strategic plan where library goals and objectives are defined. The Massachusetts Library System's (2012) two-page guide "Strategic Planning for Libraries: What It Is and Why It Is So Important" defines the strategic plan, in part, as a "living document," "a blueprint for service enhancements," and something that "helps [the] library gain recognition, funding & staffing for accomplishing the goals and objectives set out in the plan."

If the consumer health collection is to be part of an existing library, be it public, academic, or hospital or health center, the strategic plan can, of course, be modeled after and modified from the parent organization. Or it can be created. No matter the size or type of the library, there are certain elements of a strategic plan that are constant.

The Massachusetts Libraries Board of Library Commissioners (n.d.) outlines the "Parts of a Strategic Plan" (p. 11), paraphrased below:

- Mission statement: A concise declaration of the purpose of an organization, its raison d'être; identifies major service roles and user groups
- Vision statement: An uplifting and inspiring declaration of the organization's values and hopes, and what it wants to accomplish
- User needs assessment: If the consumer health library is part of a larger institution,

it might want to look at the parent institution's strategic plans to see what needs have been identified for the broader community.

Multiyear Goals and Objectives

Goals are broad statements describing desirable end results toward which the library will work over the long term, encompassing a vision of what services should be available. *Note: A goal is not measurable and may never be fully reached* (author's italics).

Objectives are specific, short-range statements of results toward a specific goal. They will define how it will be done, who will do it, and exactly how it will be done. *Note: Objectives are measurable* (author's italics).

Planning Methodology Description

This should describe the specific processes used to create the plan. If a particular process was not used, this should include a description of what was done, when the plan was developed, who participated (and to what extent), how data was gathered, and what types of data were used.

Governing Board Approval

The library's governing body must approve the plan. This could be, depending on the type of library, the board of trustees, the principal or superintendent, the dean or president, or the CEO.

Annual Action Plan Updates

The strategic plan should be reviewed annually, and an action plan should be created, listing activities that will take place the following year to achieve the strategic plan's goals and objectives.

In addition, the Massachusetts Library System (n.d.) lists several "Sample Library Strategic Plans," all from public libraries, but from communities that vary in population size from 866 at the Chilmark Free Public Library to 43,593 at the Attleboro Free Public Library, and numbers in between.

Reaching Out to Colleagues

No undertaking would be complete, however, without reaching out to colleagues. Never underestimate the value of finding out information directly from a colleague and hearing real-life experiences from those who have lived them. And if at all possible, visiting consumer health libraries would provide invaluable insights and will show what works and what doesn't.

Where to find an existing consumer health library? An excellent resource is the National Library of Medicine's MedlinePlus Consumer Health Libraries where libraries throughout the United States can be located by state (https://medlineplus.gov/libraries.html). With the information from your needs assessment and your strategic plan in hand, administration will have solid information on which to make their decision.

SPACE PLANNING

Your director or administrator or board of directors is on board and has given the "green light" to establish a consumer health collection. After appropriate and adequate celebration (with stakeholders!), the next major step is to determine and possibly create the space for your collection.

The type of library plays a major factor, be it a freestanding consumer health collection, a public library, or a library that is part of a larger institution. All have different needs and requirements, and as Stewart Brower points out, "because the potential needs and configuration of consumer health libraries can vary so widely, it is difficult to identify their common space needs" (2014, 384).

There are a number of resources to turn to. Of course, local, county, and state code and zoning laws must be followed; if the organization utilizes the services of an attorney, the attorney can help with this. If architects have been previously used, they should be consulted. In fact, depending on the size and scope of the addition, architects will have to be consulted. In hospitals and health centers, library staff will have to consult with their design and development departments.

However, no matter the type of library, certain issues apply to all. As Elizabeth Connor emphasizes, "The location and design of the library entranceway cannot be underestimated" (2011, 190). An inviting and comfortable setting is a must. The ergonomics of tables and chairs must be considered, and how many are needed. How many computers will be in the library—desktop, laptop, or both? Will there be carrels for more private study? How much shelving is necessary? This will be determined by the makeup of the collection. How many books, journals, and pamphlets will there be? And don't forget it must be accessible to all. Entrances and exits must follow Americans with Disabilities Act (ADA) guidelines, and aisles must be wide enough for customers with disabilities.

In a hospital library, the space may very well be determined and possibly limited by administration and the design and development department. This need not be an obstacle with innovative design and planning.

Space planning should be a collaborative and cooperative effort with library staff, administration, and stakeholders, using information you've discovered with your needs assessment, focus groups, and from your strategic plan.

The American Library Association has an excellent resource, *Building Libraries and Library Additions: A Selected Annotated Bibliography*. This includes the Buildings and Facilities section of the ALA online store, which quickly links to ALA's own print books, e-books, eCourses, and webinars on these subjects. And don't forget to reach out to colleagues to see what they've accomplished.

BUDGETING

The library staff should determine the amount of capital needed to establish a consumer health collection based on their needs assessment, strategic plan, and space planning. The next logical step is to create a budget. As Prottsman observes, "Libraries do not operate in vacuums. When developing the budget, the librarian must assess the needs of the organization, estimate the costs of providing resources and services to meet these needs and forecast future technological trends and environmental changes" (2011, 63).

For those who are mathematically challenged or have never had to create a workplace budget before, there is help! Cara Marcus (2014) offers an excellent overview of budgeting in her chapter "Bricks and Mortar: Costs, Budgeting, and Funding." She provides a table of "the most common budget models used in business settings" (see table 1.1).

Table 1.1. Budget Types

Name	Definition	Description	Issues and Challenges
Lump sum	A single amount of money is provided for the year to cover all the consumer health information service's financial needs. This is known as the "bottom line."	The manager is responsible for tracking and allocating funds. As long as the consumer health information service does not exceed the budget, the manager can spend on what is most needed. When the allotted amount is reached, additional spending may need to wait until the next fiscal year.	This budget is often used if a consumer health library or patient education program is considered a line under another department's budget. Accurate record-keeping is very important to justify spending and requests for additional funding.

(Continued)

Table 1.1. *(Continued)*

Name	Definition	Description	Issues and Challenges
Formula	Costs are allocated to mathematical formulas related to numbers.	An example would be estimating the interlibrary loan budget using the previous year's data of 42 articles borrowed at an average cost of $11 each, for a total of $462, and setting an ILL budget line of $500 for the next year.	This type of budget does not account for unexpected expenses, such as book replacement after flooding, or new initiatives, such as starting an eBook collection.
Line item	Each line in the budget corresponds to an object code, usually set by the finance or accounting department of the parent organization.	There may be a line for subscriptions, supplies, computer hardware, computer software, etc.	Most accounting software systems are set up for line item budgets, since other departments will consume items that can be grouped in these types of buckets. The line item budget can use a formula that takes last year's costs and applies a 7% inflation increase to create line amounts for the next year's budget. New initiatives need to be requested and approved.
Program/ performance/ function	Services associated with costs, such as document delivery, collection development, technical services, education, etc., are given lines rather than objects, such as books, brochures, magazines, etc.	Line item costs can be listed within each program/ performance/ function. Future cost estimates are based on historical data for costs in each area.	A program budget is more time-consuming and challenging to develop than a simple line item budget. It's hard to accurately determine the percentage of supplies (staples, tape, etc.) that a library will use for classes as opposed to literature packets.

Name	Definition	Description	Issues and Challenges
Zero-based	The budget is expected to remain at the same level of funding as the previous year or at a level determined by the organization.	The budget must be built from the same funding levels each year and every purchase needs to be justified.	This type of budget is one of the hardest to set up and manage, as resource costs usually increase each year, especially publications and subscriptions.
Capital	A capital budget is reserved for large physical purchases not in the regular budget, such as buildings, furniture, and computers.	This type of budget would be used to start a new consumer health information service or add new physical components. Capital requests usually have to be above a certain dollar amount and approved by senior management or the board.	As capital budgets are by nature much larger than annual operating budgets, and based on substantial one-time costs, they require coordination between many parties, such as planning committees, senior leadership, boards, development officers, architects, contractors, etc.

Of course, it is then up to the administration and the finance department to approve or modify the requests. Realistically, the requested amount always runs the chance of being rejected despite the best efforts of the library staff. Library staff should strive to work with what they are allotted, and, if necessary, seek other funding, including grants. How to fund your collection will be covered in chapter 4.

The importance of providing consumer health information to customers of all libraries cannot be understated. No small wonder that Jackie Davis (2016) very aptly titled her recent Medical Library Association (MLA) educational webinar "The Consumer Health Library: A Site for Service, Education, and Hope."

REFERENCES

Brower, Stewart M. 2014. "Physical Space in Health Sciences Libraries." In *Health Sciences Librarianship*, edited by M. Sandra Wood, 376–402. Lanham, MD: Rowman & Littlefield.

Burroughs, Catherine M., and Fred B. Wood. 2000. *Measuring the Difference: Guide to Planning and Evaluating Health Information Outreach*. National Network of Libraries of Medicine, Pacific Northwest Region (NNLM, PNR). Seattle: NNLM, PNR.

Connor, Elizabeth. 2011. "Library Space Management." In *The Medical Library Association Guide to Managing Health Care Libraries*, 2nd ed., edited by Margaret Moylan Bandy and Rosalind Farnam Dudden, 185–207. New York: Neal-Schuman.

Cuban, Sondra. 2007. *Serving New Immigrant Communities in the Library.* Westport, CT: Libraries Unlimited.

Davis, Jackie. 2016. "The Consumer Health Library: A Site for Service, Education, and Hope." Medical Library Association (MLA) webinar, April 26, 2016, 1:00 p.m.–2:30 p.m. CT.

Dettmar, Nicole. 2014. "Where to Start? Needs Assessment." In *The Medical Library Association Guide to Providing Consumer and Patient Health Information*, edited by Michele Spatz, 11–26. Lanham, MD: Rowman & Littlefield.

Institute of Medicine. 2004. *Health Literacy: A Prescription to End Confusion.* Washington, DC: National Academies Press.

Marcus, Cara. 2014. "Bricks and Mortar: Costs, Budgeting, and Funding." In *The Medical Library Association Guide to Providing Consumer and Patient Health Information*, edited by Michele Spatz, 37–56. Lanham, MD: Rowman & Littlefield.

Massachusetts Libraries Board of Library Commissioners. n.d. *Parts of a Strategic Plan.* https://mblc.state.ma.us/programs-and-support/planning/plan-parts.php.

Massachusetts Library System. 2012. *Public Library Strategic Planning: What it is and why it is so important.* http://www.masslibrarysystem.org/wp-content/uploads/Public-Library-Strategic-Planning5.pdf.

Massachusetts Library System. n.d. *Strategic Planning for Libraries: Resources & Examples.* http://guides.masslibsystem.org/c.php?g=570299&p=3930972.

McKnight, Michelynn. 2011. *The Agile Librarian's Guide to Thriving in Any Institution.* Santa Barbara, CA: Libraries Unlimited.

NCDH (Nassau County Department of Health, Division of Quality Improvement, Epidemiology, and Research). n.d. *Community Health Assessment 2014–2017.* Uniondale, NY.

Pew Research Center. 2013. *Pew Internet Health Online 2013.* http://www.pewinternet.org/files/old-media/Files/Reports/PIP_HealthOnline.pdf.

Prottsman, Mary Fran. 2011. "Financial Management." In *The Medical Library Association Guide to Managing Health Care Libraries*, 2nd ed., edited by Margaret Moylan Bandy and Rosalind Farnam Dudden, 63–78. New York: Neal-Schuman.

SCDHS (Suffolk County Department of Health Services). n.d. *Suffolk County Community Health Assessment 2014–2017.* Great River, NY.

2

Your Library's Neighborhood and Its Effects on the Health of Your Community

Takeaways from this chapter:

- *What environmental concerns affect your community*
- *How your type of community (city, suburb, rural) affects your service*
- *How to determine the specific health needs of your customers and tailor your collection to best serve them*
- *How best to reach your customers*

Libraries, especially public libraries, are situated in neighborhoods that run the gamut from poor urban to posh suburban and those whose residents can trace their ancestors back to the *Mayflower* or are themselves "fresh off the boat."

Where we live—whether it's the suburbs, the city, or in a rural area—our physical environment, the air that we breathe, the soil and flora and fauna indigenous to the area, the water supply we drink, the pollutants and contaminants distinct to our area, current health threats (e.g., mosquito-borne West Nile virus and Zika virus and scheduled open-air spraying to counter them), in short, all that defines the community's "water, air and land neighborhood infrastructure" (NCDH, n.d., 31), the climate, and the ability to access healthy food (or any food, for that matter) all deeply impact the overall health of the community.

Information on the community's specific public health concerns can be found from local (city, town, village) government and county and state government Health Departments. A complete picture of the library's community will not only help staff to tailor its collection to the specific needs of its customers, but also to know what topics to consider in community outreach and community partnerships.

Along with the community's natural environment, the "built environment is also associated with health outcomes" (NCDH, n.d., 31). Are there parks and recreational areas that not only provide opportunities for safe and healthy exercise and sports, but also for stress-reducing activities?

In addition, the library's type of community (urban, suburban, rural) will determine how customers will access the library and its consumer health resources. Is the library in a suburban setting, where personal car transportation is the norm and therefore the library has its own parking lot? Is the library in a city where the residents primarily get around using public transportation, including buses, trains, and subway, and is it an easy commute for most from home? This can be a burden for poorer customers. Or is the library in a rural setting where the library, most likely situated in the heart of the closest town, may be several miles away? In addition, some rural communities have no public transportation system.

Online collections are extremely important in today's mobile and fast-paced world and offer the opportunity for customers to access information wherever they may be. However, libraries' online access is almost always limited to library members, so the need to convey information about the library and its collections remains, including urging those eligible to get library cards.

Community demographics play a big role in determining needed consumer health resources. Residents of Suffolk County, New York (east of Nassau County, Long Island), have, like Nassau, a wide variety of incomes. At the high end are such famous areas as the Hamptons and its environs, where many wealthy celebrities own beachfront estates. Yet at the low end are areas of poverty. For example, children's exposure to lead may be a problem for some communities in Suffolk County, as "Suffolk County ranks 14th in the top 25 counties in New York State that account for 90% of lead cases" (SCDHS, n.d., p. 24). In addition, a 2016 report from the American Lung Association, part of their State of the Air 2016 initiative, "found that Suffolk County continues to have the worst air quality in the state, despite ozone levels improving."

Demographics specific to a community that are not health related per also impact on the resources needed. For example, "Suffolk County has one of the fastest growing senior citizen population rates in New York State" (SCDHS, n.d., 29); in addition, "it is estimated that 20.1% of the Suffolk County population speaks a language other than English" (SCDHS, n.d., 17). Rural areas have their own unique needs. Community Hospital-Fairfax in Fairfax, Missouri, is an eighteen-bed critical access hospital that also operates two primary care clinics. They conducted a needs assessment for the two counties they primarily serve. Holt and Atchison Counties represent 1,106 square miles in the extreme northwest corner of Missouri; the counties are rural with a combined population of 9,790. In preparing this report, Community Hospital-Fairfax conducted a community health needs assessment survey and focus groups (Community Hospital-Fairfax, 2016).

These two counties have a higher aging population than the state of Missouri, with 21 percent of the counties' population sixty-five and older compared to 13 percent for the state. The median household income is approximately $41,000, compared to the state's $53,000; more significantly, the per capita income is well below state and national averages. Both counties have less than 3 percent nonwhite populations, and less than 2 percent of households speak a language other than English (US Census Quick Facts: Atchison & Holt Counties, 2016).

Access to primary care and specialty care is a challenge in rural communities, not only because of transportation issues, but, more importantly, because of a lack of adequate numbers of area physicians. Both Atchison and Holt Counties rank near the bottom of Missouri counties for the ratio of primary care physicians to the populations. The most needed specialists were in mental health services; 35 percent of these counties' households reported depression as a problem compared to 21.8 percent of northwest Missourians, a figure similar to the state as a whole.

Residents of these counties have a slightly higher level of educational attainment than the state, with 89 percent of counties' residents possessing a high school education compared to the state's 86.3 percent. In addition, while Missouri rural residents generally have a shorter life expectancy than urban residents, for length of life these two counties rank twenty-second and nineteenth, respectively, out of Missouri's 115 counties (US Census Quick Facts: Atchison & Holt Counties, 2016).

Another type of community is Sandoval County, New Mexico, which ranks as one of New Mexico's healthiest counties, number two according to County Health Rankings and Roadmaps (http://www.countyhealthrankings.org), but has a significantly underserved section of the population. The county is 3,716 square miles, and has a population of 142,025 (https://www.census.gov), evolving from a rural and sparsely populated area in just the past decade. As the county's official website (http://www.sandovalcountynm.gov) states, it is "one of the most geographically and culturally diverse areas in the nation," and "their languages and traditions are as varied as the music and dance" of their collective cultures (Sandoval County "About").

Along with incorporated and unincorporated municipalities, the county includes all or portions of nine Indian pueblos, three Navajo chapters, and a part of the Jicarilla Apache Reservation. According to the *Sandoval County Community Health Assessment, 2015*, 90 percent of the population lives in three incorporated communities located in the southeast corner of the county (SCHC 2015).

As might be imagined, this presents obstacles to providing health and transportation services to less inhabited areas. In addition, according to the Indian Health Service, the United States Federal Health Program for American Indians and Alaska Natives (https://www.ihs.gov), American Indians continue to have lower life expectancy and a disproportionately higher disease burden compared with other Americans, due to broad quality of life issues including a history of inadequate education, disproportionate poverty, discrimination in the delivery of health services, and cultural differences.

Another part of the community of some areas are migrant and seasonal workers (e.g., farmworkers). It is often extremely difficult if not impossible for such groups to access proper health care and health information. A great source of assistance is the National Association of Community Health Centers' (http://www.nachc.org) website section on "Health Care for Migratory and Seasonal Agricultural

Workers" (http://www.nachc.org/health-center-issues/special-populations/health-care-for-farmworkers/). This lists a number of organizations to turn to, including venues and opportunities for conferences and trainings tailored to meet the needs of individuals involved in serving the agricultural worker population. Libraries might seek to be involved with providing consumer health information to this section of their communities. *And don't forget*: Any customer may suffer from "library anxiety," but those with limited formal education, those for whom English is a second language, and especially those recent immigrants who may not have had the experience of frequenting a local public library will need special attention.

While specific examples and suggestions of community partnerships and outreach programs will be covered in a later chapter, as much information as possible about who the library's customers are and how they will access the library impacts decisions about what resources are needed, and, therefore, how to budget for them.

NEED TO GO TO YOUR CUSTOMERS

According to a Pew Research Center study, *How Americans Value Public Libraries in their Communities*, "Some 81% of Americans ages 16 and older have visited a public library at one point or another in their lives, and 48% of Americans have visited a public library . . . [in the] last 12 months" (Pew Research Center 2013, 9). It's especially interesting to note that "recent library visitors are more likely to be women, those under age 65, adults who have college degrees, and adults who live in households earning $100,000 or more" (Pew Research Center 2013, 9). While library programs will, of course, be tailored to meet all library customers' interests and needs, extra efforts are necessary for specific groups.

Especially for those communities where there is a significant population of immigrants and non-English speakers, the first step for the library is to make its presence known. Where and how will you find them? This is where the library's original meetings and work with stakeholders will help.

Community centers, social and civic organizations, places of worship, and schools are just some possibilities. Is there a hospital or university in the area, or a major employer, a manufacturer or factory that employs many, if not the majority, of citizens? This would also be a place for outreach.

When the consumer health collection is in a hospital or health sciences center, the collection should first and foremost be geared toward those conditions treated and procedures done most at that institution. However, if the library is also used by patients' visitors, the collection can be expanded to include health (and preventive health) concerns that affect the community at large.

Again, community assessments will inform the library not only what issues need the most attention, but also those that would be of most interest to locals. For example, does the community have active organized sports, and if so, which ones? Information on exercising and keeping in shape would be welcome. If obesity is a major problem in the community, general information on healthy eating and healthy weight loss, as well as hints for grocery shopping and recipes, should be included.

What are the major ethnic groups in the community and which languages other than English are most spoken? Information in these specific languages should be sought and included. Keep in mind the cultural aspects of clinical care. Some cultures will not allow a male physician to examine a woman and vice versa. Some place great importance on family involvement in care and decision-making.

DISASTER INFORMATION

Some libraries are located in disaster-prone areas where hurricanes or tornadoes are a regular threat. In recent years, four US areas have seen hurricanes develop into epic "once-in-a-lifetime" events, namely, Hurricane Katrina in New Orleans, Louisiana; Superstorm Sandy in the Northeast, which devastated parts of New York and New Jersey; Hurricane Harvey in Houston, Texas; and Hurricane Maria in Puerto Rico; these hurricanes also affected other states and other island nations. And, of course, there are fires or major accidents that can plunge any area into a disaster area, not to mention acts of violence or terrorism that plague the unsettling times we live in. In August 2017, a gunman entered the Clovis-Carver Public Library in Clovis, New Mexico, a community of close to forty thousand people, and killed two employees, wounding four others. Such events have enormous physical and emotional effects on people, so the library's consumer health collection should include resources not only addressing disaster planning but also aftercare; in addition, public libraries often become a community hub when disaster strikes. And, of course, libraries need to have their own disaster plans in place for their own buildings collections and staff, as they might be directly involved.

The National Library of Medicine's Disaster Information Management Research Center, or DIMRC (https://disasterinfo.nlm.nih.gov/), is an outstanding resource for disaster information for everyone affected by a disaster, from professionals including first responders and clinicians, to community members whose homes and personal safety and health may be in danger.

To begin with, DIMRC offers the database Disaster Lit: Resource Guide for Disaster Medicine and Public Health (https://disasterlit.nlm.nih.gov/about.php); this is primarily for a professional audience. Links are provided to disaster medicine and public health documents available on the internet for free, including expert guidelines, fact sheets, websites, databases, and research reports from more than seven hundred organizations.

Libraries should sign up with DIMRC to receive their weekly updates, which provide a wealth of information on disasters. One posting alerted recipients to an online course, "Safety and Respect for All: Providing a Supportive Environment for LGBT Individuals and Families during a Disaster," and to a discussion paper, "Health Literacy Insights for Health Crises" (Parson et al. 2017), which discusses literacy-related issues concerning community messages and alerts in times of disaster. For example, if the community needs to be advised that the water supply is not safe to drink, will those with health literacy issues be able to understand documents about this?

The National Library of Medicine (NLM) offers a number of free, asynchronous, online courses on disaster health information leading to the NLM Disaster Information Specialization, both basic (Level I) and advanced (Level II). The disaster information specialization provides training to librarians and other interested professionals to support their institutions and communities throughout the disaster/emergency cycle (http://www.mlanet.org/p/cm/ld/fid=33).

Keep in mind how an area's climate will affect its residents, especially extremes in weather that will affect the citizens of different communities in different ways. Everyone may feel the brunt of blizzards and heavy snow or extreme heat and humidity; however, poorer areas are usually affected the most, resulting in a health equity issue. For example, the New York City Department of Health mapped out their most vulnerable locations during the hottest days of the year, and a dozen of those neighborhoods are in the Bronx, a borough of Manhattan. As Pereira (2017, A29) reports, "Roughly 30 percent of residents in the city's poorest neighborhoods lack air conditioning or cannot regularly use it due to high electricity costs." Libraries can make a difference and make their presence known by promoting themselves as places to cool off and enjoy health programming tailored to the needs of the patrons.

Another aspect of the community to explore are any toxic substances or pollutants that may have an impact on citizens. ToxTown (http://www.toxtown.nlm.nih.gov), also from the National Library of Medicine, is a marvelous source of information on environmental health concerns and toxic chemicals where people live, work, and play. It is available in English and Spanish. The home page is interactive, with five areas to explore: City, Farm, Port, US Southwest, and Town. After choosing one, there is a colorful picture with a variety of objects found in that area when the user rolls over the object, and the corresponding environmental health concerns are discussed; for example, the "Farm" section explores the barn and silo, vehicles, pets, and livestock. ToxTown offers information on environmental health concerns by neighborhoods, locations, and chemicals, and has an entire section for educators.

Household Products Database (https://hpd.nlm.nih.gov/) from the National Library of Medicine is a great resource for health and safety information on household products. It's next to impossible to avoid chemicals, sometimes harmful or even toxic, in everyday life. The Household Products Database allows the user to find information on products in the categories listed here with some of the products included:

- Inside the Home (bleach, cleaners, air fresheners)
- Home Maintenance (caulk, grout, insulation, paint)
- Personal Care (deodorants, hairspray, makeup, shampoo)
- Landscape/Yard (fertilizer, swimming pool products)

- Arts & Crafts (glues, glaze, varnish)
- Pet Care (flea and tick control, stain/odor remover, litter)
- Pesticides (animal repellent, insecticide, fungicide)
- Auto Products (deicer, lubricant, oil, brake fluid)
- Home Office (ink, toner, correction fluid, pens)
- Commercial/Institutional (cleaner, floor polish, lubricant)

While virtually every product will come with instructions for use and warnings, many people can't or don't read them, or don't heed them. Of course, accidents happen, and often children are involved. For example, in recent years there has been a sharp increase in children ingesting laundry detergent "pods," which can prove toxic (Valdez et al. 2014).

Sondra Cuban suggests another type of community assessment, especially in relation to the immigrant community; she calls it a "Community Asset Map." This would include "cultural asset mapping," identifying the various religious or cultural organizations and their function in the community, and how the library can work with them; "public, social, capital mapping," identifying social meeting spaces and how the library can use these as resources; and "community relationship mapping," focusing on those organizations and community leaders who can work in partnership with the library (Cuban 2007, 46–47). All these steps will enable libraries to clearly identify the consumer health needs of the community they serve.

The modern public library has become much more than a place to borrow reading materials or find information for school, although, of course, these components remain. "The vast majority of Americans ages 16 and older say that public libraries play an important role in their communities" (Pew Research Center 2013, 1). Indeed, they often act as community hubs, an anchor for the community, offering a safe, climate-controlled environment that is open long hours.

An important aspect of the library's service to the community is in providing consumer health resources. By taking a long and thoughtful look at the people in the community, their makeup, and their needs, along with the physical environment impacting them, the library staff can make the best choices for their collections. Hospital and health center libraries' consumer health collections should also be developed in concert with the needs of the parent organization's missions and the communities it serves.

It is gratifying and exciting to realize that there exists a bounty of resources for all the health needs of the library's patrons. These will be explored in the next chapter.

REFERENCES

American Lung Association. 2016. "While Nation's Air Quality Improves, Suffolk Remains Worst in State for Ozone Levels." April 20, 2016. http://www.lung.org/local-content/_content-items/about-us/media/press-releases/while-nations-air-quality.html.

Community Hospital-Fairfax. 2016. *Community Health Needs Assessment, FY 2016*. June 30, 2016. http://www.fairfaxmed.com/files/6014/6721/1573/Community_Health_Needs_Assessment_2016.pdf.

Cuban, Sondra. 2007. *Serving New Immigrant Communities in the Library*. Westport, CT: Libraries Unlimited.

Indian Health Service, the United States Federal Health Program for American Indians and Alaska Natives. https://www.ihs.gov.

NCDH (Nassau County Department of Health, Division of Quality Improvement, Epidemiology, and Research). n.d. *Community Health Assessment 2014–2017*. Uniondale, NY.

Parson, Kim, Marin P. Allen, Wilma Alvarado-Little, and Rima Rudd. 2017. "Health Literacy Insights for Health Crises." *Perspectives: Expert Voices in Health & Health Care*, July 17, 2017. National Academy of Medicine Discussion Paper. https://nam.edu/health/literacy-insights-for-health-crises/.

Pereira, Ivan. 2017. "Data: Bronx Neighborhoods Take Brunt during Hottest Days." *Newsday*, July 27, 2017, A29.

Pew Research Center. 2013. *How Americans Value Public Libraries in Their Communities*. December 11, 2013. http://libraries.pewinternet.org/2013/12/11/libraries-in-communities.

Sandoval County, New Mexico website. "About Sandoval County" http://www.sandovalcountynm.gov/about/. SCDHS (Suffolk County Department of Health Services). n.d. *Suffolk County Community Health Assessment 2014–2017*. Great River, NY.

SCHC (Sandoval County Health Council). 2015. *Sandoval County Community Health Assessment, 2015*. http://www.sandovalcountynm.gov/uploads/Downloads/Divisions/CommunityServices/HealthCouncil/SCHCCountyHealthReportFINAL.pdf.

United States Census Bureau: Quick Facts: Atchison County, Missouri. 2016. https://www.census.gov/quickfacts/fact/table/atchisoncountymissouri/PST045216.

United States Census Bureau: Quick Facts: Holt County, Missouri, 2016. https://www.census.gov/quickfacts/fact/table/holtcountymissuri/POP815216.

Valdez, Amanda L., Marcel J. Casavant, Henry A. Spiller, Thiphalak Chounthirath, et al. 2014. "Pediatric Exposure to Laundry Detergent Pods." *Pediatrics* 134, no. 6: 1–9. doi:10.1542/peds.2014-0057.

3

Building the Collection

Takeaways from this chapter:

- *Online free resources*
- *LibGuides*
- *How to write a collection development policy*
- *How to write a mission statement*
- *Online fee-based resources*
- *Print resources (books, pamphlets, and booklets), free and fee based*

The good news for all libraries is that the amount of reliable, authoritative, and readily available consumer health information, in a wide variety of formats, is absolutely amazing. Even better, much is available free. In fact, the amount of material may make collection decisions a bit overwhelming and intimidating to some librarians. However, this plethora of information should encourage librarians as they work to provide outstanding service to patrons and connect them with the appropriate information that will serve to empower them in making effective health decisions.

While there is this abundance of material, paradoxically many library patrons are not aware of its availability. Why? There are many reasons. To begin with, there is the pervasive societal mind-set that any and all health information can be provided by "Dr. Google." Of course, it's true that by using a search engine, patrons may very well find some good information, but that should not be left to chance. Other reasons vary widely based on community demographics. For example, elderly members of the community may not be in a position to utilize the library or even the internet for that matter. And many immigrant populations, both newly arrived and longtime residents, especially those who speak a language other than English, may not be aware of the library and its resources. Librarians must be proactive and help their community members find and use the wealth of information that is easily accessible.

Where to begin? While each consumer health library and collection will have its own unique needs based on the community it serves, there are some resources that can be applicable to all. The purpose of this chapter is to offer a guide to developing a core collection of resources, in a variety of formats, both free and fee based, for all libraries.

ONLINE FREE RESOURCES

It might be a surprise to some, but there is still a section of the population that has little or no experience using the internet. The library's needs assessment would determine the approximate percentage of the library's community that would be in this category. Instruction in basic internet usage is offered by many libraries and is a practice that should be implemented where needed.

The ability to navigate the internet, even in a most rudimentary way, is of great importance, if not a downright necessity, in the consumer health field. There is an abundance of online material available, and much of it is free to download in PDF format, but, for better or worse, the option to obtain hard copies in the mail is often a thing of the past.

One way libraries of all types can make this experience a little less painful for novice internet users and also generally easier to navigate for all users is to create an inviting and easy-to-understand consumer health section of their website. How to create such a website? One option is to create a site using LibGuides (https://www.springshare.com/libguides/). LibGuides is a content management platform; it is fee based according to library type or number of library patrons and also has a feature that tracks the number of views.

Innumerable examples of outstanding consumer health library collection Lib-Guides can be found on the internet. One excellent example shown is from the Mount Carmel Health Sciences Library in Columbus, Ohio (http://libguides.mccn.edu/mcchl) created by Stevo Roksandic, director. (See figure 3.1.)

Clear and attractive graphics are both appealing and functional. The consumer has no doubt where to begin and no distractions. Some customers may be overwhelmed by the home page of a website and its many options and not know where to begin.

Note that this page includes a "Medical Information Disclaimer." When a library, or any institution, provides medical information, such a disclaimer is necessary. In addition, when a library or institution directs users to other websites totally separate from its own, it's necessary for the library or institution to include some form of a disclaimer that points this out. And because patrons are seeking medical information, it's imperative that they are told that the ultimate source to answer these questions is a clinician. For example, South Nassau Communities Hospital in Oceanside,

Mount Carmel Consumer Health Information: Home

Consumer Health Information

Who needs Health Information?

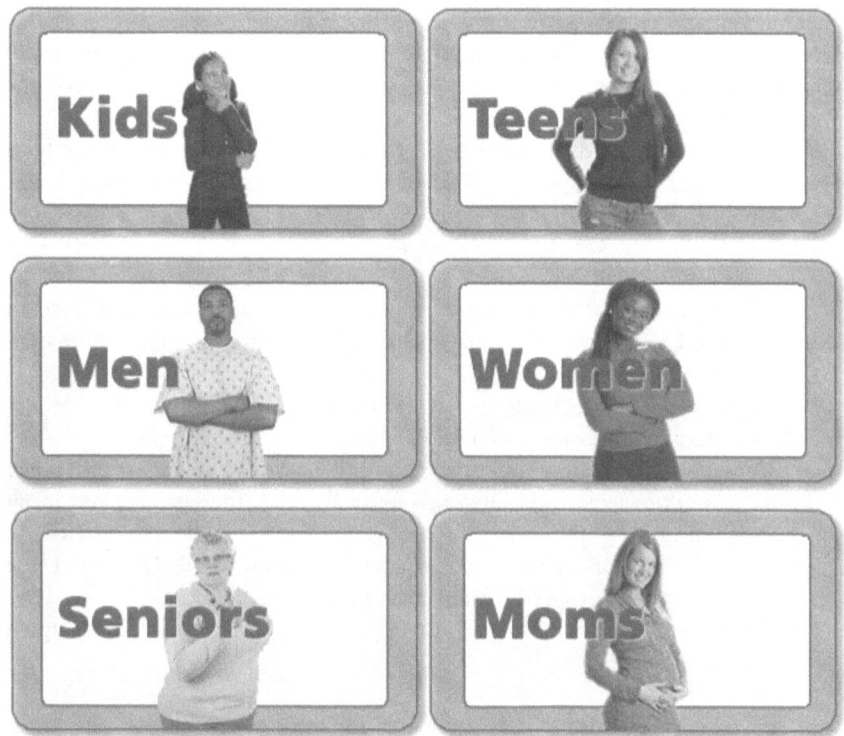

Medical Information Disclaimer

Mount Carmel Health Sciences Library (MCCHL) information that is provided in-person or accessible through MCCHL website is not an attempt to provide medical advice or professional healthcare services. Information is provided to adults for educational purposes only and is not a substitute for professional medical care or advice. We recommend customers consult their professional health care providers if they have or are concerned about any health problem or have need for any information regarding diagnosis or treatment

Figure 3.1. Mount Carmel Consumer Health Information LibGuide

New York, offers a link to MedlinePlus (http://nnlm.nih.gov/medlineplus) from their website (https://www.southnassau.org) and includes the following disclaimer:

> South Nassau Communities Hospital has not reviewed, does not endorse and is not responsible for the content of MedlinePlus or any other sites linked to MedlinePlus. Seek

the opinion of a physician for treatment or diagnosis of any medical problem, and do not rely on MedlinePlus for medical care or medical decision making. If you think you are having a medical emergency, call 911 immediately.

Of course, disclaimers should be modified to fit the circumstances of individual libraries. It might also be a surprise to some, but many internet users, even highly experienced ones, don't really know how to determine if the site they've gone to, or simply landed on, is credible. And to begin with, they don't know how to make the distinction between a search engine and a website.

The Medical Library Association (MLA) offers excellent guidelines to evaluate sites (http://www.mlanet.org/p/cm/ld/fid=398). MLA focuses on four main points, paraphrased below:

- Who is sponsoring the website?
    - The sponsor should be easily identifiable. Information should include an "About Us" profile. The site's URL ending offers additional information about the source.
    - A government agency, usually a reliable source, ends in .gov.
    - An educational institution ends in .edu.
    - A nonprofit organization ends in .org. This would include professional organizations (e.g., the American Cancer Society), foundations, and many hospitals.
    - A commercial or for-profit organization of any kind ends in .com. These sites may represent specific companies and may sell products. They need not be discounted or eliminated, but users should be clear about their purpose and intent.
- How often is the site updated?
    - The health-care field is a dynamic one, and information changes constantly. Sites should be updated frequently and offer the most up-to-date information available.
    - How often the site is updated should be clearly stated.
- Does the site present facts or opinions?
    - The site should present factual information that is capable of being verified from a primary source.
    - Opinions should be clearly stated and their source identified. Opinions need not be discounted, but they should be identified as such.
- Who is the intended audience?
    - The site should clearly state whether the information is intended for the consumer or the health professional. For websites with different sections for both the consumer and the professionals, the design should make selection of the appropriate area clear to the user.
    - Information for professionals can be highly technical, use jargon, and may be confusing, and, if not understandable, even unduly concerning to some.

These four areas can be modified to meet the needs of the library's patrons.

GETTING STARTED

The Medical Library Association's "Top Ten Consumer Health Websites" are general health sites that cover a wide variety of issues; these are highly useful for any consumer health library. They are listed below in alphabetical order, not by rank.

- Cancer.gov (http://www.cancer.gov). From the U.S. National Cancer Institute. Entire site in English and Spanish. Information includes types of cancer, treatment, and risk and prevention. LiveChat feature offers live online assistance, available in both English and Spanish.
- CDC (Centers for Disease Control and Prevention) (http://www.cdc.gov). Entire site in English and Spanish. The CDC as a source of health information is often cited by the media. While a source of highly valuable resources for clinicians, this site is also very consumer friendly. Information includes Diseases and Conditions, Healthy Living, Travelers' Health, and Emergency Preparedness. And the CDC has a mobile app available for smartphones (both iPhone or Android) with direct links to social media, text, and email.
- familydoctor.org (http://familydoctor.org/familydoctor.en.html). From the American Academy of Family Physicians. Entire site in English and Spanish. Information includes Diseases and Conditions, Prevention and Wellness, and Family Health.
- healthfinder (http://www.healthfinder.gov). From the U.S. Department of Health and Human Services. Entire site in English and Spanish. A source for consumers to "get information to help you and your loved ones stay healthy."
- HIV InSite (http://hivinsite.ucsf.edu). From the University of California, San Francisco, Center of HIV Information. "For Patients and the Public" section offers information under headings Basics, Getting Tested, Just Diagnosed, Treatment Decisions, and Living with HIV/AIDS; also includes information by Populations, including Adolescents and Youth and African Americans; a "Drug Dosing Toolkit," and a link to find services including where to get tested by city, state, or zip code.
- Kidshealth (http://kidshealth.org). From the Nemours Foundation, a not-for-profit organization devoted to improving the health of children. Entire site in English and Spanish. Separate sections for Parents, Kids, and Teens. Solid information presented in a fun and colorful way; includes movies, quizzes, recipes, and more.
- Mayo Clinic (http://www.mayohealth.org). From the venerable Mayo Clinic. "Patient Care and Health Information" section includes information on Diseases and Conditions, Symptoms, Tests, and Procedures, and Drugs and Supplements.

Be aware that the site also has links to the Mayo Clinic itself; this might be a little off putting.
- MedlinePlus (http://nnlm/nih.gov/medlineplus/). (See figure 3.2.) From the National Library of Medicine. The "gold standard" of consumer health websites. If there was only one website to access or recommend, this would be it! With one thousand health-care topics, MedlinePlus is "one-stop shopping" with information for everyone in print and video format. Entire site in English and Spanish and some information in multiple languages. Also includes an "Easy-to-Read" section. Interface is fully compatible with desktop/laptop, tablet, and cell phone.

  Note: Any library can put a link to MedlinePlus on their own site. They request that the library indicates that it is a link; complete linking instructions and restrictions can be found at https://medlineplus.gov/linking.html.
- NetWellness (http://www.netwellness.org). From three Ohio universities, offers information by topic along with sections "Research" (how to decide to participate in a clinical trial and where to find one) and a "Reference Library" that includes links to non-English websites and health information translations.
- NIH Senior Health (http://nihseniorhealth.gov). This valuable site for the "silver tsunami" of aging baby boomers is scheduled to be retired August 1, 2017. Visitors will be redirected to the National Institute on Aging's "Health & Aging" site (https://www.nia.nih.gov/health). The NIA site offers reliable and up-to-date information on health and wellness for older adults along with aging research. Links to Go4Life (https://go4life.nia.nih.gov).

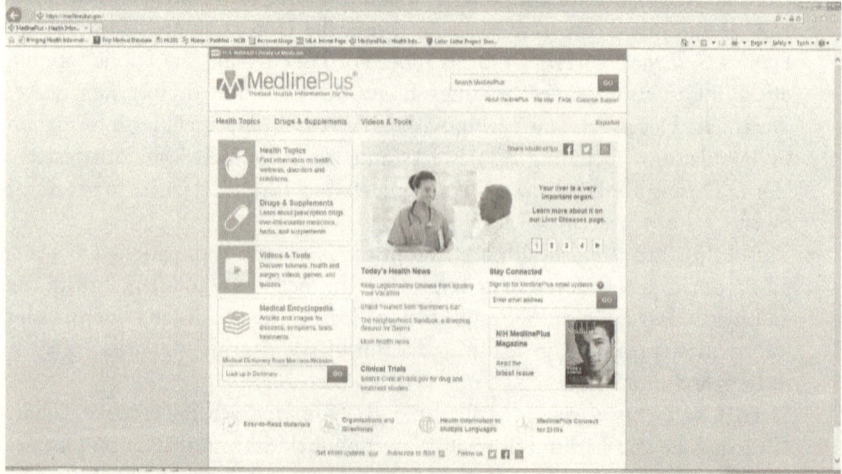

Figure 3.2.   MedlinePlus screen shot

Other websites all libraries might consider including on their "Consumer Health" page are:

- PubMed Health (https://www.ncbi.nlm.nih.gov/pubmedhealth/). This site provides information for consumers and clinicians on prevention and treatment of diseases and conditions; it specializes in reviews of clinical effectiveness research, with easy-to-read summaries for consumers along with full technical reports.
- AskMe3 (http://www.npsf.org/?page=askme3h). From the National Patient Safety Foundation. Designed by literacy experts to encourage patients and their family to ask their clinician three basic questions so they will better understand their health issue. The questions are:
  - What is my main problem?
  - What do I need to do?
  - Why is it important for me to do this?
- Lab Tests Online (http://labtestsonline.org). From the American Association for Clinical Chemistry, this site is designed to help patients and their caregivers to understand the many lab tests that are a part of health care.
- Medical dictionary. The library should certainly have one (or two) in print; online MedlinePlus provides one via a link on their home page or directly at https://medlineplus.gov/mplusdictionary.html. There is also an online visual tutorial, "Understanding Medical Words" (https://medlineplus.gov/medicalwords.html).
- ClinicalTrials.gov (https://clinicaltrials.gov). A registry and results database of publicly and privately supported clinical studies of human participants around the world. As of June 19, 2017, the site is being updated in phases to improve usability. Includes a caveat that listing on the site does not reflect endorsement by the National Institutes of Health; consumers are encouraged to consult with a trusted health-care professional before volunteering for a study.
- Genetics Home Reference: Your Guide to Understanding Genetic Conditions (http://www.ghr.nlm.nih.gov). From the National Library of Medicine, this provides consumer-friendly information about the effects of genetic variation on human health. Search for more than 1,100 health conditions, diseases, and syndromes. Resources include sections on Support and Advocacy, Financial Assistance, Genetic Testing, and Classroom Resources.
- Orphanet (http://www.orpha.net/consor/cgi-bin/index.php). The reference portal for information on rare diseases and orphan drugs (drugs intended for rare diseases), for all audiences. Includes a directory of expert resources and patient organizations.
- NLM 4 Caregivers (https://sis.nlm.nih.gov/outreach/caregivers.html). From the National Library of Medicine Outreach Activities & Resources Specialized Information Services. Includes NLM and other health resources.
- National Patient Safety Foundation (http://www.npsf.org/). Of the Institute for Healthcare Improvement. Resources for patients and families.

FOR THE K–12 CROWD AND THOSE WHO LOVE AND EDUCATE THEM

Students, educators, and health professionals, or community civic, faith-based, or recreational organizations that offer after-school programming can find all the health information they need from their regional National Network of Libraries of Medicine (NNLM). For example, the Middle Atlantic Region (MAR) offers a wide variety of resources on its website as well as in-person and online training.

One such resource list is its "Health Campaigns and Materials from Reputable Agencies" (https://nnlm.gov/mar/guides/k12-resources/materials), which is a way to learn about national campaigns and access free resources and classroom curriculums from the National Institutes of Health (NIH) and other reputable agencies. Sources include:

- Kids Health in the Classroom (Nemours Foundation) (https://classroom.kidshealth.org/). Offers educators free health-related lesson plans for all grades and subject areas. Each teacher's guide includes questions, activities, and reproducible handouts and quizzes.
- BAM! Body and Mind (CDC) (https://www.cdc.gov/bam/index.html). An online destination for kids ages nine through thirteen; very engaging and colorful, includes games.
- BAM! Teacher's Corner (CDC) (https://www.cdc.gov/bam/teachers/index.html). Provides interactive, educational, and fun activities that are linked to national education standards for science and health.
- The Brain's Inner Workings: Activities for Grades 9 through 12. From the National Institute for Mental Health (NIMH) (https://www.nimh.nih.gov/health/educational-resources/brains-inner-workings/the-brains-inner-workings-activities-for-grades-9-through-12.shtml). Multimedia resources and inquiry-based activities tied to the National Science Education Standards; includes teacher's manual and student manual.
- The Cool Spot (https://www.thecoolspot.gov). From the National Institute on Alcohol Abuse and Alcoholism (NIAAA) for kids eleven through thirteen (grades 6–8), the "young teen's place for info on alcohol and resisting peer pressure."

Genetics Resources for Students (https://nnlm.gov/mar/guides/k12-resources/genetics) includes such sites as:

- GeneEd (Genetics, Education, and Discovery) (https://geneed.nlm.nih.gov/). For students and teachers to explore all genetic-related topics; lesson plans include "Harry Potter's World: Renaissance Science, Magic, and Medicine."
- Help Me Understand Genetics (https://ghr.nlm.nih.gov/primer). Presents basic information about genetics in clear language with links to online resources.

Environmental Health and Chemistry Resources (https:nnlm.gov/mar/guides/k12-resources/chem):

- ToxMystery (https://toxmystery.nlm.nih.gov/). Grades 1–5+. Toxie the Cat helps kids find the hazards hidden in each room of the house; in English and Spanish.
- Environmental Health Student Portal (https://kidsenvirohealth.nlm.nih.gov/). Grades 6–8. Connects middle school students to environmental health information; topics include water pollution, climate change, and air pollution.
- Environmental Health Student Portal: For Teachers (https://kidsenvirohealth.nlm.nih.gov/generic/6/for-teachers). Contains links to lesson plans from a number of reputable sources.

Resources for Educators on Teen Health (https://nnlm.gov/mar/guides/k12-resources/teen-health):

- Heads Up: Real News about Drugs and Your Body (http://headsup.scholastic.com/). From Scholastic; sections for teachers, parents, kids, and administrators and librarians.
- Choose My Plate (https://www.choosemyplate.gov/). From the US Department of Agriculture (USDA). Nutrition information; sections for children, students, adults, and professionals. Available in a number of languages including Spanish, Tagalog, Hindi, Russian, and Japanese.
- Distraction.gov (https://www.nhtsa.gov/risky-driving/distracted-driving). From the National Highway Traffic Safety Administration (NHTSA). Get the facts about the consequences of texting (or allowing other distractions) while driving.

Additional Resources (https://nnlm.gov/mar/guides/k12-resources/additional):

- Profiles in Science (https://profiles.nlm.nih.gov/). Allows students to read the personal papers of Nobel Prize–winning scientists.
- *Come On, Mom, Dad, Get Healthy!* (https://sis.nlm.nih.gov/outreach/TAPAS_Mom_Dad_Get_Healthy.pdf). From the National Library of Medicine. The TAPAS (Teens Against Parent Addiction Squad) Take Action. Sixty-eight-page book is a fictional story to address addiction to food, smoking, and alcohol.

    And don't forget: Be sure to check out NNLM's *Bringing Health to the Community* blog (https://news.nnlm.gov/bhic/), which shares health information resources, news, and issues affecting communities. Categories include Children and Teens, Chronic Disease, Emergency Preparedness, Health Information Literacy, Inner City, Low Income, Minority Health Concerns, and Multilingual.
- K–12 Science and Health Education (https://sis.nlm.nih.gov/outreach/k12.html). From the National Library of Medicine Outreach Activities & Resources: Specialized Information Services. Works with teachers and scientific

experts to provide free reliable resources to help introduce, reinforce, and supplement education programs. Subjects include biology, disasters, general health, and HIV/AIDS; sections include Games, Health Information Tutorials, Lesson Plans, Projects, and Spanish-Language Resources.

COMPLEMENTARY AND ALTERNATIVE MEDICINE

According to the National Institutes of Health (NIH) National Center for Complementary and Integrative Health, approximately fifty-nine million Americans spend $30.2 billion a year out of pocket on complementary health (NIH/NCCIH 2016), so librarians need to know how to answer their patrons' questions on these topics.

Complementary medicine is defined as conventional "mainstream" medicine used together with "nonmainstream"; alternative medicine is when "nonmainstream" medicine is used in place of conventional; and integrative medicine relates to practices that bring conventional and complementary medicine together in a coordinated way.

Unfortunately many people believe that because an herb or supplement is from a "natural" source instead of from a laboratory, and does not require a prescription, it is safe to take. The reality is that herbs and supplements should be scrutinized just as carefully as any over-the-counter drug or prescription drug from a clinician. Herbs and supplements have intended effects and adverse effects along with contraindications, and consumers need to understand these factors in the same way they need to understand their prescription medications.

There are any number of reasons why consumers turn to herbs and supplements in place of or in addition to their prescription and over-the-counter medications, including mistrust of manufactured drugs and "Big Pharma" with its obscene profits, favoring "natural" products, and also cultural, ethnic, and even religious reasons.

There was a time when clinicians practicing traditional medicine frowned upon any use of herbs and supplements, but today these complementary, alternative, and integrative medications are considered acceptable under certain circumstances. The most important factor is that there must be open communication between the patient and clinician, so the patient receives the best treatment possible and avoids any dangerous combinations of drugs. For example, a consumer should not take a prescription antidepressant along with the herbal St. John's Wort.

Listed below are some excellent sources of information for the consumer health collection:

- U.S. Department of Health and Human Services, National Institutes of Health
- National Center for Complementary and Integrative Health (https://nccih.nih.gov). Outstanding source for research-based information from "acupuncture to zinc." Sections on herbs and how to find practitioners.

- MedlinePlus Herbs and Supplements (https://medlineplus.gov/druginfo/herb_All.html). Browse dietary supplements and herbal remedies and learn about their effectiveness, usual dosage, and drug interactions.
- MedlinePlus Complementary and Integrative Medicine (https://medlineplus.gov/complementaryandintegrativemedicine.html). Information on a wide variety of topics including Ayurvedic Medicine, Biofeedback, Homeopathy, Meditation, Yoga, Tai Chi, and Qi Gong; Sections specifically for children, teenagers, seniors, and women; includes videos, journal articles, and a "Find an Expert" section.
- Memorial Sloan-Kettering Cancer Center Integrative Medicine (https://www.mskcc.org/cancer-care/diagnosis-treatment/symptom-management/integrative-medicine). Consumers don't have to be current or prospective Sloan-Kettering patients to gain information from this site. Includes information on Herbs, Botanicals & Other Products; Mind-Body Therapies; and videos on "Touch Therapy for Caregivers," "Acupuncture in Cancer Care," "Guided Meditation for Relaxation and Stress Relief," and "Complementary Therapies for Pain Management."

A Note on WebMD, and Similar ".com" Consumer Health Websites

Should consumers avoid these popular sites at all cost? Is their information incorrect or biased? The answer is both yes . . . and no. Their information may be correct and helpful, but, and it's an important but, they do accept funding and advertising from, for example, drug companies. How is this a problem? One example would be if consumers assumed the only, or the best drug for their health issue, is the one advertised on the site. However, WebMD and similar sites can offer comforting connections for those who suffer from the same illness.

The 2016 sixth annual "Pulse of Online Search," conducted by Makovsky Health, a leading health-care communications company, and Kelton, a research, strategy, and design consultancy, finds that, in general, users choose sites by their familiarity and perceived ease of use, *even when they know other sites are more reliable* (author's italics).

These findings underscore the importance of advocating for reliable, trustworthy, and authoritative sources; the topic of where consumers go to find health information will be further explored in chapter 10.

And don't forget: The National Library of Medicine (NLM), the Medical Library Association (MLA), and the National Network of Libraries of Medicine (NNLM), part of the National Library of Medicine, form a powerhouse triumvirate of resources, guidance, and help for librarians seeking the best consumer health resources and outreach ideas for their communities and professional education.

NNLM is divided into eight regional areas: Middle Atlantic, Southeastern/Atlantic, Greater Midwest, Mid Continental, South Central, Pacific Northwest, Pacific

Southwest, and New England. A map (https://nnlm.gov/regions) will enable a library to determine which region it belongs to. Any library should make it a point to join its region and discover the wealth of print resources, educational opportunities, and possible funding available to it.

NNLM offers continuing education courses that librarians can use to fulfill the requirements of MLA's Consumer Health Information Specialization. Courses are taught by NNLM staff and can be conducted online, live, and/or asynchronously. Arrangements can be made for your regional instructor to offer the course in person. And they are free! These courses offer great opportunities to gain knowledge, usable resources, and networking. Recent offerings include:

- Beyond an Apple a Day: Providing Consumer Health Information at Your Library
- Health and Wellness at the Library: The Essentials of Providing Consumer Health Services
- From Snake Oil to Penicillin: Evaluating Consumer Health Information on the Internet
- The Canny Consumer: Resources for Consumer Health Decision-Making
- From Beyond our Borders: Providing Multilingual and Multicultural Health Information
- Healthy Aging at Your Library: Connecting Older Adults to Health Information
- Health on the Range: Rural Health Issues and Resources
- Locating Information on Developmental Disabilities Using National Library of Medicine Resources

COLLECTION DEVELOPMENT POLICIES

All libraries need a collection development policy. (See figure 3.3.) This will act as the library's blueprint for its collection. Many things need to be considered, including mission of the library and, for some, its parent institution. The library's community needs assessment will shine a light on the most prevalent health issues of those served; in addition, as in the case of a medical library in a hospital, the policy must be in sync not only with the mission and value statement of the hospital, but also with the major health issues presented by its patients and service lines the hospital provides. For example, if the hospital performs a high number of bariatric surgery procedures or it has a diabetes center, there should be consumer information in these areas along with general health information.

Most likely the library will want a combination of books, brochures, and other handouts; computers with lists of recommended websites; and multimedia; but in what proportions? Would the library's community much prefer print materials or websites? The mix will be determined by the information gleaned from the needs assessment.

SUBJECT: MCHSL CHL Collection Development and Management

MANUAL: MCHSL Consumer Health Library Policies & Procedures
POLICY: Collection Development and Management
RESPONSIBLE PERSONS: Library Staff

POLICY

The MCHSL CHL Collection shall include a broad range of materials to support providing accurate, timely, relevant and unbiased consumer health information needs for educational purposes only.

Priorities and limitations shall be given to materials suggested by MLA CHAPIS section, PlaneTree Health Library and Mount Carmel Health System Patient Education Department.

Literacy levels and availability of multilingual materials of the collection shall vary depending upon the profile, requirements and needs of the Mount Carmel Community.

MCHSL CHL Collection includes hard copy materials and provides access to diverse electronic accessible materials.

Hard copy materials include:

   a) books,
   b) journals,
   c) pamphlets, brochures, and other bibliographic materials.

Audio-visual materials include:

   a) DVDs
   b) CDs
   c) diverse electronic accessible materials (i.e. videos, illustration, podcasts, etc.)

Models:

   a) diverse skeletons
   b) diverse three-dimensional body parts models and sets

Electronic accessible materials are defined within MCHSL CHL Website Maintenance Policy.

Other materials shall be included into MCHSL CHL Collection if it is agreed that they support the missions, activities or programs of the MCHSL CHL.

DEVELOPED BY: Library Staff DATE: 02/07/11
REVISED BY: Library Staff
REVIEWED BY: Stevo Roksandic, Director DATE: 02/07/11
APPROVAL FOR IMPLEMENTATION BY: *Ann E. Schiele*
DATE: 02/10/11

Figure 3.3. Mount Carmel Consumer Health Library Collection Development & Management Policy

A collection policy need not be lengthy. The Collection Development & Management Policy of the Mount Carmel Health Sciences Library Consumer Health Library (http://libguides.mccn.edu/c.php?g=357643&p=2414185) is a good example of a policy that is short but one that includes all the necessary components, and its language is to the point but not so highly specific it will need to be constantly revised. The library's policy also gives an example of the standard type of format institutions use for policies and procedures.

Some highlights include:

- "The MCHSL CHL Collection shall include a broad range of materials to support providing accurate, timely, relevant and unbiased consumer health information needs for educational purposes only." "Health information needs for educational purposes only" acts as a disclaimer; nothing replaces meeting face-to-face with a clinician.
- "Literacy levels and availability of multilingual materials of the collection shall vary depending upon the profile, requirements and needs of the Mount Carmel Community." Rather than listing highly specific information, for example, stating that materials should be in English, Spanish, Arabic, Russian, Hmong, and so forth, stating instead that the languages chosen for the collection will be based on the needs of the community allows for, to put it in the vernacular, "wiggle room"; in five years the community may change in many ways, so why imbed the need to revise the policy more often than it needs to be?
- Hard copy materials include books, journals, pamphlets, brochures, and other bibliographic materials.
- Audiovisual materials include DVDs, CDs, and diverse electronic accessible materials (e.g., videos, illustration, podcasts).

This offers a broad understanding of what will be included without the need to go into highly specific explanations.

Another excellent example of a collection development policy is that of the Preston Medical Library Health Information Library, part of the University of Tennessee Graduate School of Medicine, University of Tennessee Medical Center.

SAMPLE FORM 3.1

Preston Medical Library
University of Tennessee Graduate School of Medicine
University of Tennessee Medical Center
Knoxville, TN

Health Information Center Collection Development Policy

i. The Health Information Center is co-located with University of Tennessee Graduate School of Medicine's (UTGSM) Preston Medical Library (PML) at the University of Tennessee Medical Center (UTMC). Materials are collected as part of the PML outreach mission and in alignment with UTMC's mission to serve through healing, education, and discovery. The hospital and library work together to enhance the hospital's goal of patient-centered care and educational support of patients. The Health Information Center's primary mission is to make quality consumer level health information available for patients, patient families, and area citizens. Although the Preston Medical Library maintains an assorted and diverse collection of medical resources, the Health Information Center reflects the needs of patients by focusing its collection on the hospital's Centers of Excellence and several of the major diseases of Tennessee residents. The UTMC Centers of Excellence include Brain and Spine Institute, Cancer Institute, Center for Women's and Children's Health, Emergency and Trauma Services, Advanced Orthopedics Center, and the Heart Lung Vascular Institute. The leading causes of death of Tennesseans that the collection focuses on include the following: Heart Disease, Stroke, Alzheimer's Disease, Cancer, Lung Disease, and Diabetes. The Health Information Center collection includes recent, reliable health information regarding diseases encompassed under these Centers of Excellence, other prevalent diseases, and general consumer health information. The Health Information Center does not provide interpretation of book information or interpretation of diagnoses, medical tests, treatments, symptoms, or any similar service that should be provided by a physician. Selection occurs as the center needs new materials or replaces materials. This selection policy applies to consumer health books, magazines/journals, brochures, and audiovisual resources. The Health Information Librarian is responsible for the selection of the consumer health collection. The Library Director approves the list and makes final determinations regarding any disputed materials. The center selects materials based on a combination of criteria and is in no particular order. The criteria include the following:

1. Information accuracy
2. Date of publication (generally within three years)
3. Cost of material

4. Patron and medical staff recommendations
   5. Reputation of publisher
   6. Reading level
   7. Representation of material (lack of bias)
   8. Author reliability and status in the field
   9. Application to patrons' health needs including, but not limited to
      a. Direct relation to patient needs addressed by UTMC's Centers of Excellence
      b. Direct relation to most prevalent diseases of Tennesseans
   10. For audiovisual materials, the necessary equipment to use them within the library
ii. The Health Information Center will accept gifts and donations. These items will be subject to the selection criteria above. Any gift or donation that does not meet selection criteria will be donated to another library.
iii. The Preston Medical Library seeks to maintain materials in the Health Information Center that are current and frequently circulated, and therefore reviews the collection on a yearly basis. The criteria used to determine selection is also used for collection maintenance. The Health Information Librarian provides or supervises collection maintenance.
iv. The collection will be promoted through book displays pertaining to overall patient needs, national health observances, or new materials. Librarians will also promote the consumer health collection to medical staff during library orientation so that they may encourage patients to view the collection. The library will also provide programming in collaboration with the UTMC Marketing department and during hospital sponsored medical screenings and during other events.

Updated July 2017

Unlike Mount Carmel's policy, this policy is written in a narrative style. More importantly, note that this policy uses highly specific language. The policy states that "the Health Information Center's primary mission is to make quality consumer level health information available for patients, patient families, and area citizens. Although the Preston Medical Library maintains an assorted and diverse collection of medical resources, the Health Information Center reflects the needs of patients by focusing its collection on the hospital's Centers of Excellence and several of the major diseases of Tennessee residents." The policy goes on to list the hospital's Centers of Excellence (e.g., The Brain and Spine Institute, Cancer Institute, Center for Women's and Children's Health) and also lists the leading causes of death of Tennesseans, which include heart disease, stroke, cancer, lung disease and diabetes.

They also include the all-important disclaimer "The Health Information Center does not provide interpretation of book information or interpretation of diagnoses, medical tests, treatments, symptoms, or any similar service that should be provided by a physician."

Preston's policy includes a list of selection criteria including:

- Information accuracy
- Date of publication (generally within three years)
- Reputation of publisher
- Reading level
- Representation of material (lack of bias)
- Author reliability and status in the field

Another feature of this policy is that it includes guidance on gifts and donations. This is very important, as libraries often get donation offers. While they are always well meant, and may very well be a boon to the library's collection, they can, unfortunately, include outdated materials in poor condition, donated because someone is moving or cleaning out a garage or attic.

And Preston includes an all-important section on maintenance and retention. "The Preston Medical Library seeks to maintain materials in the Health Information Center that are current and frequently circulated, and therefore reviews the collection on a yearly basis. The criteria used to determine selection is also used for collection maintenance."

Both Mount Carmel's and Preston Medical Library's Health Information Library Collection Development Policies serve as good examples to follow. They also illustrate how no two policies, just as no two libraries, will be exactly alike, and may be written in different styles, either narrative or conforming to a set policy format.

A WORD ABOUT MISSION STATEMENTS

A mission statement, quite simply, explains the library's raison d'être, answering the question "Why does this library exist?" As Finney (2008) observes, mission statements are the "cornerstone of both external communication and internal vision." They're usually short and to the point, but words must be carefully chosen to convey the message clearly. For a library that is part of a larger institution, the library's statement should reflect the mission statement of that institution.

A good example is from the Medical Library of Greenwich Hospital, which is under the leadership of Katherine Stemmer Frumento. The hospital is located in Greenwich, Connecticut, and is a 206-bed regional hospital serving Fairfield County in Connecticut and Westchester County in New York. The hospital is an affiliate of the Yale School of Medicine and a member of the Yale New Haven Health.

Their mission statement, found on the library's home page included in "About the Library" (https://www.greenwichhospital.org/medical-professionals/medical-resources/medical-library/library-services.aspx), states: "The Richard and Jonathan Sackler Medical Library's mission is to improve the medical care and research at Greenwich Hospital through the provision of resources and information, which supports patient care, clinical research, and education."

ONLINE FEE-BASED RESOURCES

There is a wide variety of fee-based consumer health online databases available to libraries. As with any resources, selection will be based on the needs assessments of the individual library, and, of course, budgetary considerations.

Fees are almost always based on the size of the institution and its potential users. In other words, vendors want to know how many users will have access to their database and charge accordingly; they usually have a formula for reaching a price. For example, if a hospital wants to pay for access to the highly regarded professional database UpToDate, the cost will be determined by (1) how many annual admissions to the hospital, and (2) how many clinicians are paid hospital employees (as opposed to "medical staff," which usually means those clinicians who have hospital privileges).

Similarly, schools, be they universities or K–12 (and everything in between), and public libraries will have similar pricing tiers or payment structures based on factors including the number of teachers and number of students, or, in the case of public libraries, community population and/or number of active cardholders. The bottom line is that the more users there are, the higher the cost. In addition, it should be noted that when dealing with major players in the industry, for example, EBSCO and Gale Cengage, "bundles" of databases are available that will bring overcall costs down. By buying several databases from these companies at one time, the library will receive better overall pricing.

Some popular fee-based databases include:

- EBSCOhost Consumer Health Complete (https://www.ebscohost.com/public/consumer-health-complete). "Informing patients on important health-related topics to foster an understanding of health." Includes full-text articles, reference

books and encyclopedias, animations, pamphlets, and leaflets on a variety of topics. One feature is information on teen health topics and how parents can learn "How to Talk to Teens" on difficult but important conversations.
- Gale Cengage Learning Health & Wellness Resource Center (http://www.gale.com/c/health-and-wellness-resource-center). Includes articles from both medical journals and general interest publications, reference works, multimedia (including streaming video), full-text reference works, and links to health-related websites.

Both EBSCO and Gale Cengage offer a wide variety of databases, and each library must determine what its users really need. For example, EBSCO also offers AltHealthWatch (https://www.ebscohost.com/academic/alt-healthwatch) for alternative and holistic approaches to health care and wellness, offering full-text articles from nearly 190 international journals.

Two other databases that should be noted:

- PubMed (https://www.ncbi.nlm.nih.gov/pubmed). The premier online database for finding research articles in the health sciences; there are more than twenty-seven million citations from biomedical literature. Because PubMed is from the National Library of Medicine, National Institutes of Health, the "basic" website is free on the internet and provides full-text access to approximately 30 percent of articles cited. As the vast majority of the articles cited are for professional clinicians and researchers, this free website should suffice for nonclinician consumers who would like to see what's in the literature on their health issue. Academic and hospital or health-center libraries might consider subscribing to PubMed Full-Text, which is a fee-based database accessible from EBSCO (https://health.ebsco.com/products/medline-with-full-text).
- CINAHL (Cumulative Index to Nursing and Allied Health Literature) is a fee-based database of nursing and allied health literature. It is available with or without access to full-text articles (the full-text version being more expensive) from EBSCO (https://health.ebsco.com/products/the-cinahl-database/allied-health-nursing).

PRINT AND MULTIMEDIA RESOURCES

What are library patrons looking to experience when they enter the section of the library devoted to consumer health? Only computers with internet access? While websites are often the best way to go, many still want to turn to print materials for their comfort level. Sium, Giuliani, and Papadakos (2015, 22) cite "three studies on the informational needs of patients and families living with cancer." They conclude that "next to extended one-on-one consults, print-based health information resources offer the most conducive context for personalized, human-to-human health communication, and satisfy patient and family needs for tangible informational tools."

It is really something of a conceit to assume that everyone has access to the internet. There may very well be in a library's community members who don't know how to access information on the internet, or may simply not have the money to buy a computer and pay for the internet access. So while the prevailing assumption may be that online health information is the current way to go, with print being not only "low tech" but also downright archaic, this is not true for the population as a whole.

BOOKS

Today's fast-paced shape-shifting internet world, combined with the highly specific needs of individual consumer health libraries, makes it difficult to come up with a "core collection" list of books. In addition, the modern acquisition standard has become, or is fast becoming, "PDA" or "patron-driven acquisition." Once again, the library should turn to the findings of its community needs assessment.

Standard resources for book selection, including *Booklist* (lj.libraryjournal.com), *Library Journal* (www.ala.org/offices/publishing/booklist), *Kirkus Reviews* (www.kirkusreviews.com), *Publisher's Weekly* (www.publishersweekly.com), book dealers, and vendors are all resources for consumer health texts. The Consumer and Patient Health Information Section (CAPHIS) of the Medical Library Association regularly reviews books in its newsletter, *Consumer Connections*. Issues are available at CAPHIS's section of the MLA website. Some publishers that are of interest include:

- Childhood Cancer Guides (https://www.childhoodcancerguides.org) are wonderful sources to help families of children with cancer.
- Hilton Publishing (www.hiltonpub.com/publishing/hilton-books/) offers a variety of consumer-health-related books. (Another division of the company publishes Patient Direct Educational Materials for patient discharge and take-home summaries on hundreds of topics in English and Spanish.)

And don't forget: Any consumer health library might consider a good medical dictionary and an anatomy textbook for starters.

PHYSICIAN DIRECTORIES

Thanks in no small part to the internet, we live in an increasingly consumer-oriented society. At one point in our history, clinicians' decisions and advice went unquestioned, but today's consumer is not only more than willing to challenge clinicians, but also seeks "ratings" for them, for both professional qualifications and expertise and also overall clinician-patient experience (e.g., friendliness of staff, wait to see the clinician, waiting room condition).

For questions regarding physicians' qualifications, professional experience, and to check to see if there are any malpractice issues regarding them, the patron must turn to the internet.

MedlinePlus offers sections on "Organizations and Directories." Directories include the AMA Physician Select: Online Doctor Finder; DocInfo from the Federation of State Medical Boards of the United States; Medicare Physician Compare; and a list of professional medical organizations to "Find Doctors by Specialties." Also included is a section on "Other Healthcare Providers," including the HRSA (Health Resources and Services Administration) Find a Health Center and a list of specialized hospitals and clinics.

State licensing bureaus offer valuable information on physicians; for example, in New York State the "New York State Physician Profile," at https://nydoctorprofile.com—information is available in English and four other languages and includes the physicians' educational background and any legal actions taken against them.

PAMPHLETS AND BOOKLETS

Health-related associations and organizations offer a wide variety of pamphlets or booklet-type materials for consumer health patrons and patients, items that they can take home and keep. Unfortunately, many are only available as free PDF downloads, so library staff may need to print them out for their customers. However, there are still a number of print copies available free of charge.

Some sources include:

- *MedlinePlus Magazine* (https://medlineplus.gov/magazine/). This excellent magazine is available both online as a PDF and in print; bulk quantities can be ordered free of charge. Cover stories link celebrities with health issues; recent issues include cover stories on singer Nick Jonas and type 1 diabetes; Olympic swimmer Michael Phelps dealing with depression; actress Kathy Bates living with lymphedema, and former NFL quarterback Doug Flutie on "Sports and Concussion." There is also a Spanish version, *MedlinePlus Salud* (https://medlineplus.gov/spanish/magazine/). This is published less frequently and features Latino celebrities and their health issues.
- FDA (Food and Drug Administration) (https://fda/gov/forconsumers/) has a number of informative health fact sheets and brochures for Children, Women, Minority Health, Health Educators and Students, and Patients; they must be downloaded. Many are offered in multiple languages including Arabic, Bengali, Chamorro, French, French Creole, Tagalog, Urdu, and Polish.
- National Institute of Dental and Craniofacial Research (NIDCR) (https://catalog.nidcr.nih.gov/OrderPublications/) offers a number of free publications on all types of dental issues for all ages; some are in Spanish. All are available for download; many are available in print.

- The National Institute of Mental Health (https://www.nimh.nih.gov/health/publications/index.shtml). A wide variety of mental health issues are covered in both English and Spanish. All are free for download; some are available in print.
- Nutrition.gov (https://www.nutrition.gov). Free source of information on food and nutrition from the National Agricultural Library, USDA. Wide variety of topics covered for different age groups in English and Spanish. All are free for download; some available in print.
- *Stroke Connection* magazine (http://strokeconnection.strokeassociation.org/). Magazine from the American Stroke Association. Can be read as a PDF or ordered in print.

Fee Based

- Channing Bete (www.channing-bete.com) offers a wide variety of products for consumers and professionals alike, including many consumer/patient handouts for "readers of all ages, cultural background, and reading levels). In general, prices are low with quantity discounts.
- Journeyworks (http://www.journeyworks.com). Health promotion and health education pamphlets; low cost (especially in bulk) and easy to read; multicultural and Spanish pamphlets also available.
- Krames Patient Education (https://kramesstore.com). Educational booklets and videos for patient education and discharge, but may be useful for all consumer and health collections.

GRAPHIC NOVELS AND COMICS

Yes, graphic novels and comics! Their popularity is wide ranging and inclusive, and their easy-to-read format makes them credible resources for a library's consumer health collection, and one that should be seriously considered; as Buono says, "Respect comics even if you don't like them" (2013, 159).

In fact, the 2017 Comics and Medicine Conference, an annual conference of Graphic Medicine (http://www.graphicmedicine.org) held at the Seattle (Washington) Central Library, was funded by NNLM Pacific Northwest Region (PNR) with a $12,000 grant; keynote speaker events were free to the public. The 2017 conference theme was "Access Points"; comics can be considered "accessible" as they reach diverse audiences and can provide a platform for marginalized voices, and they "can make visible and reflect upon the urgent subject of health access" (Long 2017).

Matthew Noe, graphic medicine specialist at NNLM New England Region (NER), suggests (2017) that one important reason to include comics is the fact that comics are "a medium that has mass appeal, can convey complex subjects in simple ways, and can cross any number of barriers to access."

NNLM NER offers "Graphic Medicine Book Club Kits" to any New England–based organization (Connecticut, Maine, Massachusetts, New Hampshire, Rhode Island, and Vermont) free of charge. Each kit includes six copies of a graphic novel, a quick guide to reading comics, discussion questions, and topic-relevant MedlinePlus information. Kits are offered in the following (NNLM NER, n.d.):

- Topic: Addiction
  - Title: *Sobriety: A Graphic Novel* by Daniel Maurer (2014)
  - Description: From the publisher . . . "Through rich illustration and narrative, *Sobriety: A Graphic Novel* offers an inside look into recovery from the perspectives of five Twelve Step group members, each with a unique set of addictions, philosophies, struggles, and successes while working the Steps."
- Topic: Aging
  - Title: *Can't We Talk about Something More Pleasant?* by Roz Chast (2014)
  - Description: From the publisher . . . "Roz Chast and her parents were practitioners of denial: if you don't ever think about death, it will never happen. *Can't We Talk about Something More Pleasant?* is the story of an only child watching her parents age well into their nineties and die. In this account, longtime *New Yorker* cartoonist Chast combines drawings with family photos and documents, chronicling that 'long good-bye.'"
- Topic: AIDS
  - Title: *Pedro & Me: Friendship, Loss, & What I Learned* by Judd Winick (2009)
  - Description: From the publisher . . . "Pedro Zamora changed lives. When the HIV-positive AIDS educator appeared on MTV's *The Real World: San Francisco*, he taught millions of viewers about being gay and living with AIDS. Pedro's roommate on the show was Judd Winick, a cartoonist from Long Island, and the two soon became close friends. Judd created *Pedro and Me* to honor Pedro Zamora, his friend and teacher, and most of all, an unforgettable human being."
- Topic: Cancer
  - Title: *Mom's Cancer* by Brian Fies (2006)
  - Description: From the publisher . . . "*Mom's Cancer* is a graphic novel about one family's struggle with metastatic lung cancer. Honest, unflinching, and sometimes humorous, it is a look at the practical and emotional effect that serious illness can have on patients and their families. In the end, it is a story of hope—uniquely told in words and illustrations."
- Topic: Epilepsy
  - Title: *Epileptic* by David B. (2005)
  - Description: "A painfully honest examination of the effects of debilitating epilepsy on one man and his family, told through a combination of straightforward text and expressionist imagery that ranges in its palette from centuries-old symbolism to the secret worlds of childhood. Even as he shows up the hollow promises of every school of esoteric and alternative medicine

his family encounters in their quest for help, David B. works a real kind of deeply human magic on the page—something forged from black ink and a soul's struggle—that marks *Epileptic* as one of the first truly great narrative artworks of the new millennium."—Jason Lutes

- Topic: Grief
  - Title: *Rosalie Lightning* by Tom Hart (2016)
  - Description: From the publisher . . . "*Rosalie Lightning* is Eisner-nominated cartoonist Tom Hart's beautiful and touching graphic memoir about the untimely death of his young daughter, Rosalie. Hart uses the graphic form to articulate his and his wife's ongoing search for meaning in the aftermath of Rosalie's death, exploring themes of grief, hopelessness, rebirth, and eventually finding hope again."
- Topic: LGBTQ
  - Title: *Fun Home* by Alison Bechdel (2006)
  - Description: "At once a coming-out story, an examination of the complex relationship we can have with our parents and the role of art and literature in processing our lives. . . . Smart, darkly funny and a little fearless, *Fun Home* reads like a true-life modern American Gothic."—*Time* Best Comics of 2006
- Topic: Mental Health
  - Title: *Marbles: Mania, Depression, Michelangelo, and Me* by Ellen Forney (2012)
  - Description: From the publisher . . . "Shortly before her thirtieth birthday, Ellen Forney was diagnosed with bipolar disorder. Flagrantly manic but terrified that medications would cause her to lose her creativity and livelihood, she began a years-long struggle to find mental stability without losing herself or her passion. With dazzling storytelling, bold illustrations, and razor-sharp wit, *Marbles* offers a wholly unique and visceral glimpse into the effects of a mood disorder on an artist's work and seeks to answer: IS mental illness a curse, or is it actually a gift?"
- Topic: OCD/Doctor-as-Patient
  - Title: *The Bad Doctor* by Ian Williams (2015)
  - Description: From the publisher . . . "Meet Dr. Iwan James: cyclist, doctor, would-be lover, former heavy metal fan, and, above all, human being. Weighed down by his responsibilities—from diagnosing personality disorders to deciding who can hold a gun license—he doubts his ability to make decisions about the lives of others when he may need more than a little help himself. Cartoonist and Doctor Ian Williams introduces us to Iwan's troubled life as all humanity, it seems, passes through his surgery doors."
- Topic: Veteran's Health (This Kit is unique in that it contains two titles)
  - Title: *At War with Yourself* by Samuel Williams (2016)
  - Description: From the publisher . . . "In this illustrated conversation between Samuel C. Williams and his friend, Matt, they talk candidly about Matt's struggles with post-traumatic stress disorder. From scoping out quick exits

in coffee shops to re-experiencing his traumatic events, Matt describes his unique experiences and how he has learnt to cope."
- Title: *When I Returned* from the Center for Cartoon Studies (2016)
- Description: "*When I Returned* is a comics anthology containing six unique stories from veterans at the White River Junction VA Medical Center in Vermont. Illustrated by a number of cartoonists from The Center for Cartoon Studies, these stories help show the depth and variety of the 'veteran experience.'"

Fotonovelas are similar to comic books, but instead of drawings, photographs are used. They are a traditional print medium and immensely popular in Mexico, Latin America, and the Caribbean. Libraries should consider obtaining or even creating their own fotonovelas on various health topics of special importance to their community; in fact, their inclusion would be a great way to attract new immigrants to the library (Houston 2013, 151). And a library working in partnership with a hospital or health center in creating fotonovelas would be a wonderful consumer health initiative.

A number of health-related organizations offer a very limited number of fotonovelas, so be sure to check their websites for these items. For example, the Environmental Protection Agency (EPA) has a fotonovela in English and in Spanish for an introduction to their Toxic Release Inventory (TRI). These provide invaluable information regarding the toxic chemicals found in the community. These TRI fotonovelas are only available as slideshows or as PDFs for download (https://www.epa.gov/toxics-release-inventory-tri-program/tri-fotonovela-latinohispanic-novella-style-introduction-tri).

The Rural Women's Health Project (RWHP) offers fotonovelas on a variety of health topics, in English and in Spanish, at nominal cost. Topics include abuse, smoking, contraception, and pregnancy (http://www.rwhp.org/catalog/).

The absolute wealth of consumer health information is exciting. Library staff will find it a "labor of love" to connect resources with patrons, as there is great satisfaction, both professionally and personally, in helping patrons become empowered regarding their health.

REFERENCES

Buono, Michael. 2013. "Reaching Out through Graphic Novels." In *Library Service for Multicultural Patrons: Strategies to Encourage Library Use*, edited by Carol Smallwood and Kim Becnel, 157–61. Lanham, MD: Scarecrow Press.

Finney, Christopher. 2008. "Mission Haiku: The Poetry of Mission Statements." *NonProfit Quarterly*, March 5, 2008. https://nonprofitquarterly.org/2008/03/05/mission-haiku-the-poetry-of-mission-statements-2/.

Houston, Cynthia. 2013. "Fotonovelas and Historietas: Adult Comic Books from Mexico in American Libraries." In *Library Service for Multicultural Patrons: Strategies to Encourage*

Library Use, edited by Carol Smallwood and Kim Becnel, 149–56. Lanham, MD: Scarecrow Press.

Long, Thomas Lawrence. 2017. "CFP: 2017 Comics & Medicine Conference: Access Points." Literature, Medicine, & Medical Humanities: An MLA Commons site. January 19, 2017. https://medicalhumanities.mla.hcommons.org/2017/01/19/cfp-2017-comics-medicine-conference-access-points/.

National Institutes of Health. National Center for Complementary and Integrative Health 2016. *Americans Spend $30 Billion a Year Out-of-Pocket on Complementary Health Approaches*. https://nccih.gov/research/results/spotlight/americans-spend-billions.

National Institutes of Health. National Center for Complementary and Integrative Health. https://nccih.nih.gov.

NNLM NER (National Network of Libraries of Medicine New England Region). n.d. "Graphic Medicine Book Club Kits." https://nnlm.gov/ner/guides/graphic-medicine-book-club-kits.

Noe, Matthew Nicholas. 2017. "Consumer Health: Comics in the Medical Library." *MLA News*, July 17, 2017. http://www.mlanet.org/p/cm/ld/fid=1122&&blogaid=1606.

Sackler Medical Library, Greenwich Hospital, *Mission Statement*. https://www/greenwichhospital.org/medical-professionals/medical-resources/medical-library/library-services.aspx.

Sium, Aman, Meredith Giulani, and Janet Papadakos. 2015. "The Persistence of the Pamphlet: On the Continued Relevance of the Health Information Pamphlet in the Digital Age." *Journal of Cancer Education*, November 18, 2015. doi:10.1007/s13187-015-0948-3.

Sixth Annual Makovsky/Kelton *Pulse of Online Search Survey*. 2016. http://www.makovsky.com/news/makovsky-pulse-of-online-search-survey-2016/.

South Nassau Communities Hospital. https://www.southnassau.org.

4
Grants

Takeaways from this chapter:

- *How to find funding*
- *How to apply for grants; grant proposal writing*

After careful planning, preparation, and collection development, the library is now ready to start purchasing books, journals, computers, furniture, and everything else that it will need to provide the best possible consumer health collection for its clients. There's just one all-important item needed: funds to pursue these goals.

When it comes to funding, libraries may face a number of obstacles. Perhaps the library's administration has indeed earmarked funds in the budget specifically for the consumer health collection, but it might not be enough for everything and especially not enough to pursue outreach projects. Or perhaps the library's administration has approved an annual budget for the next year but, when that year arrives, requires a certain percentage of the budget be cut. Or perhaps the library's administration finds the idea of a consumer health collection or project a worthy and admirable pursuit, but for a variety of reasons either cannot or will not provide adequate funding.

Resourceful librarians will not let lack of funding or not enough funding stop them from pursuing their goals. It's now time to look for and pursue appropriate grants. Even in tough economic times there is money to be had, but there is competition for limited funding. So where and how to start?

GRANT PLANNING

By this time, the library has performed a detailed community needs assessment and has not only identified the makeup of community customers and their specific health needs, but has also connected with community stakeholders and laid the groundwork for partnerships.

Take all this information and brainstorm with staff and community stakeholders. Community stakeholders may very well be a source of grant funding resources, including local civic and community groups and local companies, those both privately held and those that are branches of national corporations. Be sure to zero in on areas where there is a strong community health need. For example, does the community have a large immigrant population or a large senior population? What are the health issues of the community?

Once a plan for a collection or community outreach has been determined, the next step is to find a grant from an organization whose requirements closely match the needs of your program. An application for an ill-fitting grant is a waste of precious time for both the library and the granter. Whether it's for the library's collection development or a library outreach project, alone or in a partnership, the plan must have a clear vision with a reachable goal and a measurable outcome.

Simply stating "We need money and our administration won't give it to us" may be the unvarnished truth, but it will never result in winning any grants. In addition, broad or vague requests, for example, "Our library wants to start a consumer health collection," will also not suffice. A specific plan for consumer health information that will in some way, shape, or form improve the health of the community that the library serves must be identified, described, and explained.

One of the best places to begin the quest for funding for consumer health programs is the National Library of Medicine's National Network of Libraries of Medicine (https://nnlm.gov/). One of NNLM's goals is to improve public health through access to health information.

Eight regional medical libraries provide a variety of outreach services, and member libraries include academic health sciences libraries, hospital and health sciences libraries, public libraries, and community-based organizations.

The regional medical libraries are divided into state grouping. For example, the Middle Atlantic Region (MAR) serves Delaware, New Jersey, New York, and Pennsylvania, while the Greater Midwest Region serves Illinois, Indiana, Iowa, Kentucky, Michigan, Minnesota, Ohio, North and South Dakota, and Wisconsin. Every US state is covered by a region, so the first item of business is to reach out to the library's region, although chances are good that the regional staff has already reached out to the library.

The NNLM regional websites also provide information on programs that have been funded. Some recent initiatives that have been funded by NNLM/MAR (https://nnlm.gov/mar/funding/funded) include:

- Queens (NY) Library Mobile Health Information Classroom (https://nnlm.gov/mar/funding/funded/5517). Superstorm Sandy had a devastating effect on the residents of Far Rockaway, New York, and two public libraries in the bor-

ough of Queens were severely damaged. With this $10,000 award, the Queens Library was able to purchase technology and offer health information services within mobile units.
- Health Information on the Go: Reaching Rural Populations by Bookmobile (https://nnlm.gov/mar/funding/funded/6217). The Columbia County (NY) Traveling Library does community outreach in partnership with area agencies. With this $15,000 award, this ongoing initiative seeks to outfit a new bookmobile as a mobile classroom to reach rural populations that experience significant health and economic disparities. Their "goals are to create awareness about MedlinePlus and other quality consumer health information resources, increase their use, and connect people to local resources and services which will improve health and quality of life."
- Promoting Health Literacy by Training Front-Line Staff in a Hospital Setting (https://nnlm.gov/mar/funding/funded/6222). Wilkes-Barre General Hospital (WBGH) is located in Luzerne County, Pennsylvania, which is higher than average in indications of a population at risk, including the age of the population and poverty. As the largest hospital in the area, WGBH "has a huge impact on the health of the community." With this $15,000 award, this ongoing initiative "will be used to increase knowledge of health literacy among the health professionals on staff through training" and will also provide access to "materials to support health literacy training and patient/consumer health and resource awareness."
- Cooking for Good Health and Happiness 2015 (https://nnlm.gov/mar/funding/funded/6071). The Laurel (DE) Public Library received a $3,000 award to continue a popular interactive program that introduces older adults to healthy cooking techniques and free online health information resources, "focusing on what is available through MedlinePlus and NIHSenior Health."

Woodson and Timm (2016, 67) describe the LSU (Louisiana State University) Health Shreveport Health Sciences Library faculty's "successful and ongoing project to emphasize wellness issues for preschoolers in a creative manner. To accomplish this, the librarians offered health-related story times with follow-up activities at locations within the community." With funding from the National Network of Libraries of Medicine South Central Region (NNLM SCR) and partnership with the local public library system, the Shreve Memorial Library, this innovative and creative community outreach program strives to educate young children on healthy eating to avoid overweight and obesity and its related health conditions including hypertension and type 2 diabetes. One activity they developed is the grocery bag game, which takes children on an imaginary adventure to the grocery store and distinguishes between healthy and unhealthy food choices.

It is always a good idea to peruse programs that have been successful in winning grants as this will not only give you further indications about what the funding organization is looking for but also colleagues to reach out to.

In addition to NNLM regional networks, there is a wide variety of funding sources, including federal, state, and local governments; private organizations; and community service groups.

Other Grant Funding Sources

The Foundation Center (http://foundationcenter.org) is the leading source of information on grants, and their main focus is to connect nonprofits with grant opportunities:

- The Foundation Directory itself is an online database that requires a subscription (http://foundationcenter.org/products/foundation-directory-online).
- The Foundation Directory Online Quick Start (http://foundationcenter.org/find-funding/fdo-quick-start) provides free access to information on more than one hundred thousand foundations.
- The Foundation Center recently launched "Visualizing Funding for Libraries" (http://libraries.foundationcenter.org), "the most comprehensive free database of library funding that has ever existed."

Other grant sources include:

- The United Way (http://www.unitedwaynca.org/pages/members-grants), which offers Community Impact grants to invest in specific community-centered issues.
- Funding Information Networks, in all fifty states; the center's Grant Space Find Us page (http://grantspace.org/find-us) will locate an area resource center.

Federal

Check out the Institute of Museum and Library Services (IMLS) (www.imls.gov). The mission of IMLS is to inspire libraries and museums to advance innovation, lifelong learning, and cultural and civic engagement.

The US Department of Education (www2.ed.gov/about/contacts/state/index.html) provides a nationwide list of state contacts including the Department of Education and the Adult Education agencies.

And speaking of states, don't forget the state's Health Department. For example, the New York State Health Department (https://www.health.ny.gov/funding/) lists all current grants and funding opportunities and information on the grant, application forms, and due dates.

A great place to start would be by approaching the federal and state government elected officials who would most likely be delighted to champion the library's search for funding for programs that would improve the health of the community they all serve. Elected officials should also have knowledge of funding sources and opportunities.

And don't forget: If the consumer health library is part of a larger institution, a hospital, or an academic center, find out if there is a grants department, and/or a community education or outreach department; the library may be able to partner with them for a project. If the consumer health library is in a public library, reach out to the local hospital or health center; there may be a partnership possibility.

GRANT WRITING

Writing a grant can be a lengthy and daunting process that needs great attention to detail and precise and complete fulfillment of all application requirements.

And application requirements can be quite involved and quite lengthy. An application for a "Community Health Outreach" Award from NNLM Pacific Northwest Region (NNLM PNR) is eight pages long and requires the following information:

- Project title
- Proposed start and end dates for the project
- Summary statement: a one-paragraph summary of the project's goals and objectives, the intended outcomes, and the work plan
- Description of the target audiences and need for the project
- The goals of the proposed project
- The specific objectives to be achieved by the project; objectives should be stated in measurable terms.
- A detailed work plan (max one thousand words) and a rationale for the plan
- Evaluation plan: explain how the success of the project will be measured and the methods to measure that success
- A timeline for the project
- Identification of all project personnel and their role in the project
- A list of types of partner organizations the library will work with to carry out the project
- Names, addresses, websites, and descriptions of partner organizations and key contacts
- A budget plan form, which should be accompanied by a narrative justification to provide sufficient supporting detail
- Forms identifying direct beneficiaries/populations targeted
- Form identifying NNLM goals that apply

Also required are (1) curriculum vitae of key personnel and (2) letters of support from the applicant's institution. These letters might include one from the CEO, and one from the head of IT if technology is involved.

A required cover sheet with specific information is also needed. In addition, applicants should include a cover letter. Once the application has been completed in its entirety, the applicant will have a better understanding of how to approach the cover letter. General rules of writing a good cover letter apply. The goal is to write a professional appeal for the grant summarizing in one page the needs for the grant and its goals and objectives.

Grant Writing Assistance

Hospitals and health sciences libraries connected to large health centers or universities are sure to have a grants department, and any library grant will need collaboration with them. In fact, most likely the library staff will provide the information and the grants writer will actually write it. The organization's department of external affairs, community relations, or community outreach (or whatever title the organization has given to it) may also need to be involved.

For those libraries that do not have a staff grants writer to turn to, there are sources of guidance. NNLM offers information on "Proposal Writing Support" (https://nnlm.gov/funding/support) that includes "Grant/Proposal Writing Tips and Tutorials," along with additional funding resources and MLA and NNLM classes on grant writing; NNLM staff may be able to provide online or in-person training on "Grants and Proposal Writing" if the library has the need and time for this (and enough of an audience). In addition, NNLM's "Developing a Program: Planning and Evaluation Methods/Grant and Proposal Writing" (https://nnlm.gov/mar/guides/proposal-writing) provides links to a Community Tool Box, "Getting Grants and Financial Resources," and to the Foundation Center's "Proposal Writing Short Course," a free online self-paced course.

The Purdue University OWL (Online Writing Lab) offers some general guidance on grant writing (https://owl.english.purdue.edu/owl/resource/981/1/).

Gerding and MacKellar (2017, 133–38) offer the following "Tips for Grant Success" that apply to all grant seekers:

1. Focus on people.
2. Plan ahead.
3. Know what you want to accomplish.
4. Meet community needs.
5. Be realistic.
6. Ask for what you need.
7. Actively engage.
8. Partner and collaborate.
9. Be positive.
10. Pay attention to the details.
11. Be persistent.

Another source for assistance in grant writing is Reed and Nawalinski's (2016) *Getting Grants in Your Community*, a publication of United for Libraries, the Association of Library Trustees, Advocates, Friends, and Foundation, a division of

ALA. This was updated in 2016 for "Books for Babies" funding, but the guidance given will work for all kinds of proposals and all types of libraries. In the section "Finding the Money," they suggest doing some "homework," and finding out all the possible funding sources in your area, including civic groups (Lions Club, Rotary, the Junior League, etc.), local businesses, local corporations, and community foundations. When working with a "big box" store, for example, Target, the library must investigate the company's policy and history of giving to the community. As Quelch, Koh, and Yatsko (2016) point out, some large companies want to address community health challenges not only to improve the health of citizens, including their workforce, but also to strengthen their corporate social responsibility strategy.

Finding a suitable grant and applying for it is a lot of work, but winning a grant can give a library the means of reaching its goal of providing the best consumer health information or program to its community that has the power to make a difference in the health and well-being of that community.

REFERENCES

Gerding, Stephanie K., and Pamela H. MacKellar. 2017. *Winning Grants: A How-to-Do-It Manual for Librarians*. 2nd ed. Chicago: Neal-Schuman.

Quelch, John, Howard Koh, and Pamela Yatsko. 2016. "Why Companies Like IBM, Target and LL Bean Invest in Community Health." *Forbes*, October 18, 2016. https://www.forbes.com/sites/hbsworkingknowledge/2016/10/18/why-companies-like-ibm-target-and-l-l-bean-invest-in-community-health/#3f8418171489.

National Network of Libraries of Medicine/Middle Atlantic Region (NNLM/MAR). *Past Funded Projects*. https://nnlm.gov/mar/funding/funded.

Reed, Sally Gardner, and Beth Nawalinski. 2016. *Getting Grants in Your Communities*. Bryn Mawr, PA: United for Libraries. http://www.ala.org/united/sites/ala.org.united/files/content/products_services/booksforbabies/toolkit/getting_grants_book.pdf.

Woodson, Deidra, and Donna F. Timm. 2016. "Rewards and Challenges of Children's Health Education: An Ongoing Community Partnership to Reach Local Preschoolers." In *Consumer Health Information Services and Programs: Best Practices*, edited by M. Sandra Wood, 67–86. Lanham, MD: Rowman & Littlefield.

5

Staff Customer Service

Takeaways from this chapter:

- *Customer service training for all staff (volunteers, professionals)*
- *Specific customer service training for consumer health libraries*

The old adage "You only get one chance to make a first impression" rings true whenever people meet. Yes, it is sometimes possible to "redo" or mitigate bad first impressions depending on the circumstances, but, in general, the opportunity to do this might just not happen. The goal of consumer health library staff (or any library staff for that matter) is to provide a good first impression that will then naturally lead to excellent customer service.

Especially in today's mobile and social media world, where so many exchanges are made online, including via texting (even when participants are physically in the same space!), it is more important than ever to ensure that all staff knows how to greet people and make them feel welcome and comfortable.

While good customer service should be considered quite simply the right thing to do, as it is a way of showing respect and interest for patrons and their informational needs, developing and practicing good customer service has the added professional perquisite of shining the spotlight on just how much skilled librarians are needed. With the prolific use of the internet and the pervasive mind-set that all information can be found by searching Google unassisted, some administrators are closing health sciences libraries and eliminating librarian positions. We can heed Bernstein's words, "How do we as librarians ensure that we and our libraries do not become obsolete? I believe the question can be answered in two words: customer service" (2008, 21).

As Shipman and Lake pointedly observe, "If you've seen one consumer library, you have seen one consumer library." No two libraries will have the exact same needs.

Staffing is influenced by location, hours of operation, library mission, and services. "The one thing that is constant among consumer libraries is that staff is the most important resource" (2014, 77). This chapter will focus on those magical two words, "customer service."

While each consumer library is unique, there are basic good customer service practices that are the same for all libraries, if not all places of business. For any library, organization, or business, a customer's first experience with a staff member can often "make or break their library's success" (Shipman and Lake 2014, 77). Staff represent the institution as a whole; they are the embodiment of the library. If service is good, the customer will return and share good "ratings" with friends and family, but if service is bad, the customer will be reluctant at best to return and will convey their displeasure to others. And poor customer service is not limited to active "bad behavior" on the part of staff; a customer can easily receive bad service by neglect. Not greeting customers or "ignoring" them is just as bad as cranky behavior.

Many customers seeking consumer health information are in a uniquely vulnerable position as they are seeking answers to health-care questions for themselves or loved ones that may very well be "life or death." Add to this the fact that customers may be intimidated by the library and its staff in general as they may rarely if ever use libraries, have no idea where to look for information or even how to ask for it, may be elderly, may speak a language other than English, may have problems with literacy, or may have some combination of all these factors. So consumer health library staff must be trained to be particularly sensitive to how they treat their customers. Staff should be visible, approachable, and friendly. Libraries should adopt the business rule for customer engagement, the "10-5 Rule" (or the similar "10-4 Rule"):

- *When staff is within ten feet of a customer, make friendly eye contact and smile.*
- *When staff is within five feet (or four feet) of a customer, speak to the person in a friendly tone of voice that conveys approachability and invites the customer to begin a dialogue. Note: A simple "Good Morning" will do.*

Everyone can relate to the frustration they feel after making eye contact with someone only to have that person look away! And remember how it feels when waiting in line in a store while the clerk finishes his or her private conversation.

If staff members are busy helping another customer, they can quickly and easily acknowledge the new patron by simply saying "Hello" or "I'll be with you in a minute," or asking another staff member to jump in.

Carr makes an excellent point when he states that "the first step in refining your library's customer service attitude starts with your users—both current users and potential users. We need to take a snapshot of what the customers' expectations might be" (2013, 116). The consumer health library can determine this not only with the extensive needs assessment they've developed, but also with the very nature of this specialized collection, the content of which will be tailored to the community's needs. Consumer health library customers will be seeking health information that can run the gamut from exercise and diet information all the way to understanding the possibly devastating illness of themselves or a loved one and what can be done about it.

Consumer health libraries, like any other library or institution, have to develop customer service training that is mandatory for every employee. If the library is part of a health sciences center, or college or university, there will be employee information required of all new employees regardless of their position. For example, hospitals require all new employees to attend organizational orientations that describe hospital-wide policies and procedures that affect everyone, including standards for safety and infection control. Certainly all libraries will have general expectations of all of their employees. And each and every position, from volunteers to professional librarians, must have a specific job description that includes in detail everything that is expected of the holder of that position.

LIBRARIANS

The Medical Library Association's "Professional Competencies for Health Sciences Librarians" (http://www.mlanet.org/p/cm/ld/fid=39) is a good resource. The American Library Association's "Core Competences of Librarianship" is a good starting point, but as ALA notes, "Librarians working in school, academic, public, special, and governmental libraries, and in other contexts will need to possess specialized knowledge beyond that specified here" (ALA 2009, 1).

However, as Shipman and Lake point out, "Where do librarians for a consumer library come from? Do they have to be medical librarians or have experience working in a health sciences library to be effective? Surprisingly, no" (2014, 79). Not only hospital and health sciences librarians qualify for the job, but also public librarians who possess easily transferable skills, including the ability to work successfully with a diverse public with widely ranging informational needs and educational achievement.

For those librarians outside the health sciences or hospital world, training in consumer health sources is readily available. NNLM regional libraries offer in-person training classes and information on nationally available NNLM training opportunities; training is often given online and asynchronously. For example, check NNLM's Middle Atlantic Region (MAR) page (https://nnlm.gov/professional-development). The Medical Library Association offers a "Consumer Health Information Specialization" (http://www.mlanet.org/p/cm/ld/fid=329). Basic and advanced training opportunities are available for those whose work roles demand that they provide consumer health information services to the public, patients, and families.

And along with their culture of service, librarians are also collegial and are always willing to "cross over" from one type of library to another to help each other. One need not look too far for examples of just such cooperative efforts. In Oklahoma, a state that ranks poorly on multiple measures of health and wellness, health sciences librarians and faculty librarians from the Robert M. Bird Library (BHSL) at the University of Oklahoma Health Sciences Center (OUHSC) created a "collaborative network of health information professionals in Oklahoma's public libraries through the implementation of the Health Information Specialists Program" (Clifton et al. 2017, 254). This program was designed to provide continuing education and networking opportunities for public library staff who are interested in consumer health resources and services (Clifton et al. 2017, 255). Courses were approved for the Medical Library Association for credit toward the Consumer Health Information Specialization. The authors conclude that the program had a positive impact on the health information expertise of those public librarians who participated, resulting in increased consumer health information knowledge to be passed on to their patrons.

Another such initiative was the Virginia Commonwealth Libraries Tompkins-McCaw Library for the Health Sciences (TML) where staff librarians developed a series of classes aimed at public, hospital, and health sciences librarians (Ladd and Hurst 2017). They received funding from the NNLM Southeastern/Atlantic Region (SEA) to be used to offer the class series in a free two-day workshop titled "Providing Consumer Health Information to Patrons: A Workshop for Librarians." Attendees can receive up to ten hours of continuing education credit from the Medical Library Association, which are approved for credit toward the Consumer Health Information Specialization. And not only is the workshop free, mileage, parking, and a one-night hotel accommodation will also be provided!

VOLUNTEER STAFF

Volunteers can be quite a diverse group of people depending on their community and the type of library they work in. Their ages can run from teenage to elderly, and their skills will be wide and varied. In a hospital setting, volunteers will either state what type of work they're interested in, or be given a list of positions and departments that need volunteer help. In public libraries, volunteers may be interested residents, or may be fulfilling community service requirements, be they court ordered or, for many teenagers, accomplishments needed for their college applications. Each library will have its own policies and procedures regarding volunteers. In a hospital setting, volunteers will receive orientation about hospital-wide policies and procedures and will be required to have health clearance before they can begin work.

When a professional librarian is available, volunteers can be limited to greeting patrons and, if the question is simple and straightforward (e.g., "Do you have material on diets?"), to point the patron in the direction of material or a computer offering premade lists of websites. More complex questions should always go to the librarian, who has training in not only the reference interview, which may include "teasing" out the real question the patron needs answered but also where and how to find best information.

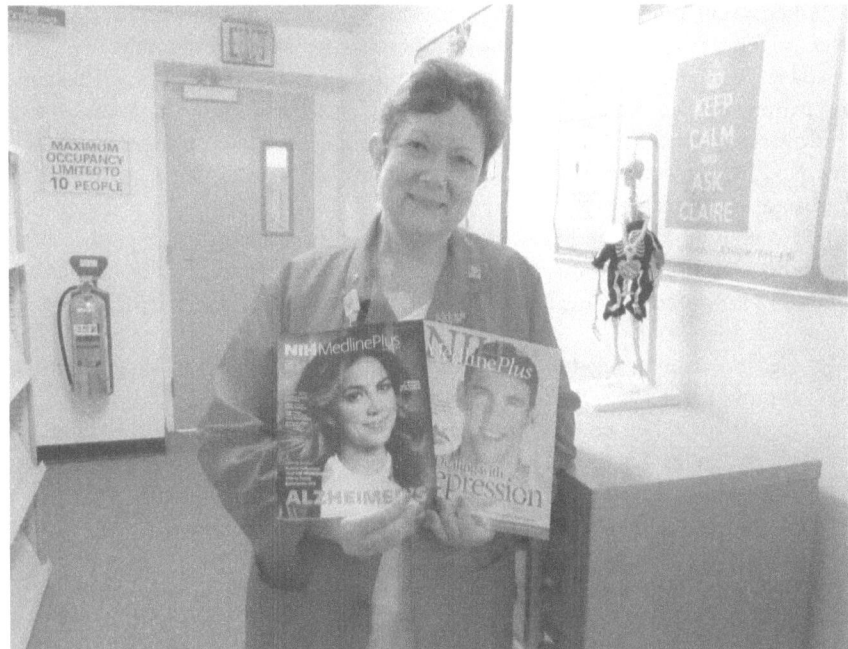

Figure 5.1. Volunteer ready to serve
Courtesy of Sue Keller

Some health center libraries provide information service for patients and visitors. At the Brigham and Women's Faulkner Hospital Patient/Family Resource Center (P/FRC), "volunteers provide door-to-door service by delivering health information and books to patrons" (Marcus 2016, 9). (See figure 5.1.)

CUSTOMER SERVICE SKILLS FOR ALL STAFF

The University Library at the University of Illinois at Urbana has developed GREAT Customer Service Guidelines (http://www.library.illinois.edu/administration/services/great.html). They break down to:

G   Greet all customers and make them feel welcomed
R   Respect cultural and other personal differences
E   Evaluate and clarify customer's needs
A   Address and respond to customer's needs
T   Thank and verify that needs have been met

All library staff should make a personal and library-wide commitment to inclusiveness and cultural competency in collections, programs, and customer service.

Library staff must learn that an important part of good customer service is to treat all patrons in an open, friendly, and nonjudgmental way or manner. The staff members' personal ideology must not come into play. For example, staff will encounter patrons who are seeking information on such hot-button topics as abortion and euthanasia. And staff must greet all customers in the same way, regardless of ethnicity, race, gender, or identifiable religion (e.g., woman wearing hijab, man wearing turban or yarmulke).

Of course, library staff members are people with their own thoughts, beliefs, prejudices, and so forth, and no one is beyond an occasional blunder or misstep. This is where proper training comes in. Staff members should be given the following:

- General training regarding the mission and purpose of their library and the community it serves
- Review of skill set needed for the staff member's specific position and duties (of course, the new hires will have been screened to ensure they possess such skills, but it's imperative that they are aware of all their job requirements)
- Sensitivity training regarding treating all people whom the staff member will encounter
- Regular continuing education training to ensure customer service continues to be great

The library should consider designing and implementing an inclusive staff training program. Kowalsky and Woodruff (2017, 65–67) speak specifically of patrons with disabilities, but the ideas they set forth would apply not only to those with disabilities but also multicultural, multiethnic, and the LGBTQ communities.

In both group discussions and self-awareness exercises that can be done at home, employees should be encouraged to reflect on personal biases, preconceived ideas, feelings, and attitudes towards "others," groups outside of themselves. It would be a great idea to involve members of the library's multiethnic, multicultural, and LGBTQ community to assist with the training. Role-playing—creating realistic scenarios with staff playing both patrons and staff—are often very effective methods of raising staff's understanding of situations and patrons they may encounter. Reach out to organizations who often provide sensitivity training. For example, the Long Island LGBT Network (http://www.lgbtnetwork.org) offers workshops and training at the workplace. Community leaders of civic, cultural, or religious organizations should be invited to speak to employees, and it could be arranged for employees to visit houses of worship or cultural organizational events. In addition, the library should seek to participate in community events such as street fairs. The library can set up its own table complete with staff members (especially librarians) and a sampling of the consumer health information that is available at the library. And the librarians at the table need to be proactive and say hello to anyone that goes past the table; don't wait for people to come to the table. Perhaps a relatively inexpensive item might be raffled off, and remember that candy always attracts people!

Of equal importance in customer service is culturally competent staff training; such training should be customized to the library's community. Members of the community, especially community leaders representing the major cultural groups, or, in some cases, the myriad of cultures in the area, should be invited to address library staff to educate them on that group's culture and norms to raise cultural awareness.

Staff should be encouraged to reflect on their own cultural background, norms, and biases, and conduct role-playing exercises to deal with cultural conflicts. Staff should also be educated to realize that some immigrants may come from areas where the US concept of a public library is unknown to them, and many rules of library use, including the (in some libraries) requirement for quiet and fines for overdue books may also be concepts that need to be learned (Cuban 2007, 131–32).

CULTURAL HUMILITY

The Nassau Queens Performing Provider System (http://www.nq-pps.org), an alliance of three major health systems located in Nassau and Queens Counties, New York, offers a Cultural Competency and Health Literacy training webinar, presented by Martine Hackett, PhD. The author "attended" this as a member of her hospital's Cultural Initiatives Committee. Dr. Hackett in her training, uses, along with the term "cultural competency," the term *"cultural humility"* (author's italics), certainly an outlook and attitude that libraries can emulate and embrace in their customer training and service.

And don't forget: When a library patron asks for assistance, personally escort the person to the area of the library where the information can be found, be it the computer station or a bookshelf. The hospital where the author works has instructed all staff (a "nonnegotiable" directive) to personally escort visitors to where they need to go; in other words, if a visitor asks a passing staff member where a certain department or area is, the staff member should not just give directions, for example, "Walk down this hall, turn left, turn right," and so forth. Escort your customers to where they want to go. This personal touch, whether it's in a hospital, library, or anywhere for that matter, makes a huge difference in service. And all consumer health library staff should be passionate—or at least enthusiastic—about the very special service they're providing to their customers. In addition, staff should never overlook their *internal* customers, their fellow staff members. All the customer service skill practices should extend to everyone.

The library profession has always been, is, and will continue to be service oriented, yet Buono asserts that "good customer service is rare. . . . Cultural barriers that prevent easy communication can often fluster even experienced librarians. When people become flustered, the tenets of good customer service break down" (2013, 303). All libraries should educate staff and put policies in place that create a culture of acceptance and inclusiveness for all library patrons. Without good customer service, vital resources and information will be underutilized or unused, and the mission of the library will be unfulfilled.

REFERENCES

ALA (American Library Association). 2009. "Core Competences of Librarianship." http://www.ala.org/educationcareers/sites/ala.org.educationcareers/files/content/careers/corecomp/corecompetences/finalcorecompstat09.pdf.

Bernstein, Mark P. 2008. "Am I Obsolete? How Customer Service Principles Ensure the Library's Relevance." *AALL Spectrum* 13, no. 2: 20–22.

Buono, Michael. 2013. "Risk Looking Stupid." In *Library Service for Multicultural Patrons: Patrons: Strategies to Encourage Library Use*, edited by Carol Smallwood and Kim Becnel, 303–7. Lanham, MD: Scarecrow Press.

Carr, Steven. 2013. "Refining the Customer Service Attitude." In *Staff Development: A Practical Guide*, 4th ed., edited by Andrea Wigbels Stewart, Carlette Washington-Hoagland, and Carol T. Zsulya, 113–25. Chicago: American Library Association.

Clifton, Shari, Phill Jo, Jean Marie Longo, and Tara Malone. 2017. "Cultivating a Community of Practice: The Evolution of a Health Information Specialists Program for Public Librarians." *Journal of the Medical Library Association* 105, no. 3: 254–61. doi:dx.doi.org/10.5195/jmla.2017.83.

Cuban, Sondra. 2007. *Serving New Immigrant Communities in the Library*. Westport, CT: Libraries Unlimited.

Kowalsky, Michelle, and John Woodruff. 2017. *Creating Inclusive Library Environments: A Planning Guide for Serving Patrons with Disabilities*. Chicago: American Library Association.

Ladd, Dana L., and Emily J. Hurst. 2017. "A Consumer Health Workshop for Librarians." *CAPHIS Consumer Connections* 33, no. 2 (April): n.p.

Marcus, Cara. 2016. "A Most ResourceFULL Consumer Health Information Center." In *Consumer Health Information Services and Programs*, edited by M. Sandra Wood, 1–18. Lanham, MD: Rowman & Littlefield.

Shipman, Jean, and Erica Lake. 2014. "Prized Assets: Staff." In *The Medical Library Association Guide to Providing Consumer and Patient Health Information*, edited by Michele Spatz, 77–95. Lanham, MD: Rowman & Littlefield.

6

Library Privacy and Confidentiality

Takeaways from this chapter:

- *What degree of privacy and confidentiality of patrons is required by the library*
- *How to determine what level of privacy and confidentiality patrons would like and how to provide it*

Librarians have a long, proud, and documented history of promoting and protecting their patrons' intellectual freedom rights to access information in a way that ensures their privacy and confidentiality.

But in today's world, how much privacy can we offer patrons with health-related questions, and what actions can we take to ensure this? What expectation of privacy do patrons have? We must be sure to find this out and offer it. While privacy and confidentiality is always our goal, providing privacy can be quite challenging at times. Librarians must find just the right mix of common sense, compassion, and professional training to ensure that we have made every attempt to meet patron expectations.

CONFIDENTIALITY AND PRIVACY

Confidentiality

While the terms "confidentiality" and "privacy" are used somewhat interchangeably in some circumstances, for the purposes of this chapter patron privacy will be understood to mean asking for and/or accessing information without observation or without being overheard; patron confidentiality will be understood to mean keeping any and all individually identifiable information secret.

When writing policy statements, confidentiality can be defined, while a definition of privacy is somewhat difficult to nail down. According to American Library Association (ALA) standards, confidentiality refers to anything that specifically identifies an individual. For example, what patrons check out is confidential and requires a court order to access. After the horrific events of September 11, 2001, the ensuing enactment of the US Patriot Act placed some libraries in an ethical quagmire as they were asked to provide just such records in an attempt to find terrorist-related activities. According to ALA's (2005) "Confidentiality and Coping with Law Enforcement Inquiries: Guidelines for the Library and Its Staff," "Without a court order, neither the FBI nor local law enforcement has authority to compel cooperation with an investigation or require answers to questions, other than the name and address of the person speaking to the agent or officer." And in ALA's (n.d.) "Questions and Answers on Privacy and Confidentiality," they advise that "if a librarian is compelled to release information, further breaches of patron confidentiality will be minimized if the librarian personally retrieves the requested information and supplies it to the law enforcement agency. Otherwise, allowing the law enforcement agency to perform its own retrieval may compromise confidential information that is not subject to the current request."

The American Library Association has a wonderful resource, their "Privacy Tool Kit" (http://www.ala.org/advocacy/privacy/toolkit), that covers every aspect of how a library can protect the privacy of its patrons. Sections include:

- Privacy and Confidentiality: Library Core Values
  - Covers Privacy and the Law, Standard Privacy Principles, and PII (Personally Identifiable Information)
- Developing or Revising a Privacy Policy
  - A Privacy Audit and Sections to Include in a Privacy Policy
- Implementation of Privacy Policies and Procedures
  - Responsibilities of Governance Bodies/Policy Makers
  - Responsibilities of Directors/Supervisors
  - Responsibilities of Staff
  - Library Policy Talking Points: Key Messages and Tough Questions
    - Key Messages
    - Tough Questions with Answers
  - What Is ALA Doing
  - Advocacy at the Local, State & National Levels

Every library should have a privacy policy, which, for all intents and purposes, is really speaking to customer confidentiality. The New York Public Library (2016) has ninety-two locations including four research centers and a network of neighborhood libraries throughout Manhattan, the Bronx, and Staten Island. They serve some eighteen million patrons annually, and their website receives thirty-two million visits annually from more than two hundred countries. Yet the concerns of their privacy policy (https://www.nypl.org/help/about-nypl/legal-notices/privacy-policy)—which is freely available on their website to print, email, or share, and is also in Spanish, Russian, and Chinese—are the concerns of any library. Their lengthy policy covers what individually identifiable information they collect (e.g., residence, social media information, personal use of circulating and noncirculating materials, Internet Protocol [IP] address, location, websites visited) and how they use this information. It is a good example of all the issues a library must confront regarding privacy; however, not every library must have such a lengthy policy! Each library must decide what is necessary to include in its policy.

And every patron who uses a "third-party library services provider," for example, a database, should be informed that simply by logging on they may provide information directly to the third party. Suffice it to say that it is incumbent on every library to provide the best internet security (virus protection, firewalls, etc.) that is available and to deal with only reputable third-party vendors who can substantiate their online security protocols.

Privacy

Privacy, or providing both a space to ask questions and accessing information without being observed, can be a little more problematic, especially in today's internet/social media world and especially with the ubiquitous cell phone. Most cell phone users have little or no expectation of privacy; in fact, it sometimes seems that some users want to be sure their phone conversations are overheard.

For internet use, privacy screens are the answer. Privacy screens are relatively inexpensive, removable, and available for monitors, laptops, tablets, and even smartphones. They are readily available from both library supply and office supply firms. If they are not already installed on library computers, they should be offered and available for use. These give patrons the ability to access health information in private and also offer protection from hackers.

For face-to-face interactions between librarian and patron, privacy may be difficult, but it must be offered. Health issues are highly personal and may be fraught with emotion. It is incumbent on librarians to first ascertain the level of privacy the patron desires and then make every effort to deliver it.

The Medical Library Association and the National Network of Libraries of Medicine (NNLM) offer valuable guidance in not only providing privacy, but also in establishing a comfortable atmosphere for the patron. In addition, guidance is also offered regarding the ethics of providing health information.

With regard to privacy, the NNLM's (n.d.) "The Consumer Health Reference Interview and Ethical Issues" advises that the librarian be mindful that "because of the personal, sensitive nature of health topics, consumers may be reluctant to approach the library staff member. Use welcoming behaviors like making eye contact, smiling, and greeting the patron," the latter, of course, being advice to follow for any librarian in any library. In addition, NNLM advises that a library "provide a private area to discuss confidential topics. If there is not adequate privacy at the reference desk, take the person to the book stacks, an office, or another quiet area. Lower your voice if needed to maintain privacy, and assure the patron that confidentiality will be maintained. Do not discuss any reference interactions with other staff members, unless professional expertise is needed to answer the question." And the Medical Library Association (MLA 2010), in its "Code of Ethics for Health Sciences Librarianship," advises that "the health sciences librarian respects the privacy of clients and protects the confidentiality of the client relationship."

Health questions present unique ethical considerations that librarians must remain mindful of. NNLM offers a good summary checklist of ethical considerations, adapted from Healthnet: Connecticut Consumer Health Information Network:

1. Provide a welcoming, safe environment.
2. Be aware of the person asking the questions, but don't make assumptions.
3. Get as much information as possible.
4. Verify medical terminology in a medical dictionary or encyclopedia.
5. Be aware of the limitations of medical information.
6. Provide the most complete information to answer the information request.
7. Do not interpret medical information or provide advice.
8. Provide referrals.

Remember, a consultation with even the best librarian can never take the place of a consultation with a trained clinician. However, the information librarians provide patrons can be invaluable and provide patrons with solid knowledge of their health issue and better understanding of how to work with their clinicians, what questions to ask them, or even where to find a clinician that can best help them.

We know that every library should have a policy statement on privacy and confidentiality, and certainly a consumer health library can follow the guidelines of the ALA, NLM, and MLA. But how does a library successfully put these goals into practice?

ON THE FRONT LINES OF CONSUMER HEALTH SERVICE

Privacy, in the modern library, is highly problematic, so depending on the library and its location, consumer health librarians must be especially sensitive to ensuring the highest possible private, safe, and welcoming environment for their patrons.

Academic, health center, and hospital libraries remain, for the most part, true to the conventional stricture of keeping libraries quiet, with patrons using their "indoor voices," as they are usually used as places of often intense study.

Public libraries, on the other hand, have long since discarded the enforcement of quiet; in fact, many are quite noisy places. Reference librarians generally sit in a visible and open setting, so for those who answer a significant number of consumer health questions, a more private location should be available, especially for highly sensitive questions. And, again, in today's culture of ubiquitous cell phone conversations, the concept of privacy has changed significantly, and is many times nonexistent.

Patrons may not have any expectation of privacy. They may approach a librarian and ask questions, even highly personal and sensitive ones, making no attempt to speak quietly, with full knowledge that there are any number of people nearby.

Nevertheless, it is always incumbent on the librarian to inquire of patrons if they would like to continue the discussion in a more private place. It should also be noted that whatever literature the librarian finds for the patron should be offered privately.

LIBRARIAN-PATRON REFERENCE SCENARIOS

Scenario I

A nurse comes to her hospital's medical library looking for information to help manage her teenage son's bipolar disorder; his condition has taken an alarming turn, as he has begun to lash out physically in anger and the nurse is worried what will happen.

As a health-care professional and, more importantly, a mother, this nurse has explored and investigated her son's condition, and he has seen and continues to see specialists and receives treatment. However, the nurse reaches out to the librarian in the hope that the librarian, as an information professional, could find specialists, programs, and schools that the nurse cannot find on her own.

In addition, the nurse asks the librarian to perform a literature search to find the latest theories and therapies regarding her son's disorder. Of course, this is all highly personal information. Yet the nurse has no problem initiating a conversation with the librarian while she is at her desk, which is out in the open, and with full knowledge that there are other patrons in the library. In addition, the nurse has a loud speaking voice.

The librarian, at the beginning of the conversation, asks the nurse if she would like to discuss this someplace else where it is more private. The nurse declines. The librarian searches for local specialists and programs. She remembers that a colleague, a psychologist who has often asked her for the latest updates on bipolar disorder, might very well know of a specialist in their area. She reaches out to him, keeping the identity of the nurse confidential; in fact, she does not even mention that her patron is a staff nurse.

When the librarian has completed her searching, she prints out all the information and places it in an interoffice envelope that she personally delivers to the nurse. In this instance, the librarian has provided a degree of privacy to the best of her abilities.

Scenario II

A community member has just learned that her mother has stage IV cancer, a life-threatening diagnosis that has seemingly "come out of the blue," as symptoms that had been assumed to be benign have instead proven to be an indication of just how far this deadly disease has progressed. She is beside herself, not thinking straight, but she decides to go to the public library and find out if the prognosis for her mother is, indeed, a dire one. She would also like to find specialists to consult. This trip to the library is a highly personal journey and one that is fraught with insecurities and fears.

As she approaches the reference desk, she realizes that any conversation she would have with a librarian would be very much out in the open with no privacy. She is about to leave when a librarian greets her and asks if she can be of help.

The researcher burst into tears and blurts out that her mother just got a diagnosis of inoperable cancer. The librarian gets up, takes the patron aside, and says, "Come with me; we can talk about this in a more private place." She takes the patron to one of the library's quiet rooms where she speaks to her in a low voice.

The patron is then able to collect herself and ask the librarian how she can find out about this cancer, its prognosis, and specialists to treat it. The librarian is happy to assist her and has provided her patron with the privacy she sought.

EMPLOYEE TRAINING IN PRIVACY

Consumer health collections can run the gamut of a few dedicated shelves or bookcases of materials in an existing library to freestanding consumer health libraries.

Those serving patrons may be volunteers, clerical staff, highly trained professional health sciences librarians, or combinations thereof. Some hospitals and academic medical centers have imbedded or clinical librarians that may actually access patients' records via their electronic medical record (also called electronic health record). The latter is an exception to the rule, as hospital employees are usually only permitted to access patients' health records if they are directly involved with that patient's care, so the employee is usually a clinician.

All places of employment give their new hires some form of employee orientation. In large institutions such as a hospital, that orientation can last an entire week or more. In smaller institutions, orientations are often one-on-one between a department head and the new employee. Every institution has policies and procedures manuals, and all employees are made aware of them. Libraries' privacy and confidentiality policies must be included in orientation.

From the volunteer who simply directs a patron to the consumer health section to the professional who assists a patron in finding understandable answers to complex questions, ethical considerations of privacy must be upheld.

All libraries provide consumer health information in some way, shape, or form. Librarians and other library staff members must be mindful that health-related questions are some of the most difficult and personal to ask. With ethical and professional guidelines in place, library staff must offer a welcoming environment and whatever level of privacy their patron desires. The bottom line is making sure that patrons receive the best information available and have their questions answered with sensitivity and compassion.

SAMPLE FORM 6.1

The New York Public Library Privacy Policy

Last Updated: November 30, 2016

Privacy is essential to the exercise of free speech, free thought, and free association. The New York Public Library ("NYPL" or "Library") is committed to protecting your privacy, whether you are a user, visitor, and/or donor. This Privacy Policy explains what information we collect from you and why. By using our website, downloading our mobile applications, visiting a Library location, or donating to us, you agree to this policy. You also agree to let us use your email and postal address to communicate with you about our programs, services, fundraising efforts, and more. While New York State law requires that we treat as confidential information about materials you check out and information you access (NY CPLR Section 4509), we also do so because it is in keeping with our commitment to you to protect your privacy. In developing this Privacy Policy, we drew upon industry best practices and national standards for privacy.

This Privacy Policy may change from time to time by posting such changes to our website, so we encourage you to check back periodically for updates. We will alert you to material changes that have been made by indicating on the policy the date it was last updated, by placing a notice on our website, by sending you an email and/or by some other means.

What information does NYPL collect?

We collect information about you in three ways: directly from you, from automatically collected network logs, and through cookies. We typically keep information only for so long as it is needed for the proper operation of the Library and in order to better deliver Library services to you. We may retain some information in backup storage systems, hard copy form, or as required by law. We collect different types of information from you depending on your chosen level of engagement with our Library services and the information needed in order to provide you with access to those services.

1. ***User-Provided Information.*** When you register for a user account for our Library services, we may ask you to share certain information with us. If you register with us, we offer you the opportunity to review and, when practical, to update, change or delete some information you have provided us. You can do this by logging into your registered user account or you can ask our staff to assist you by phone at 1-917-ASK-NYPL, or by emailing us at gethelp@nypl.org, or by visiting a Library location and speaking to our staff. If you deactivate your registered user account, you may not be

able to continue using certain Library services that require registration. The following are examples of information that you might be asked to provide to us:

- **Personal Information**: any information that can personally identify you, such as your name, physical address, email address, phone number, Library barcode, payment information, and other similar information.
- **Residency Verification**: information such as driver's license, other government-issued identification, and utility bills containing a postal address (click here for a complete list of acceptable forms of proof of residency).
- **Shared Content**: includes anything created by you that you choose to make public by using our Library services. Your registered user account and any information you have chosen to display may accompany your shared content.
- **Social Media Information**: includes the option of using your social media accounts and posting content on our social media pages, our crowdsourcing sites, or elsewhere on the Internet, and such information you allow to be shared with us.
- **Login Credentials**: includes username, password, and a set of personal questions about you and are provided as part of the process to create an online user account which allows you to view your Library Records at any time by logging into your account.
- **Library Record**: contains your Personal Information related to your personal use of circulating and non-circulating Library materials, including but not limited to computer database searches, interlibrary-loan transactions, reference queries, e-mails, faxes, requests for photocopies of Library materials, title reserve requests, and the use of audio-visual materials such as films and music.

We are committed to keeping such information, outlined in all the examples above, only as long as needed in order to provide Library services.

2. *Information NYPL Automatically Collects.* When you use our Library services, such as our website and mobile applications, our computer servers automatically capture and save information electronically about your usage of our Library services. Examples of information that we may collect include:

- Your Internet Protocol (IP) address
- Your location
- Kind of web browser or electronic device that you use
- Date and time of your visit
- Website that you visited immediately before arriving at our website
- Pages that you viewed on our website
- Certain searches/queries that you conducted

If you are using a Library device, we may also record your Library barcode, time and length of your session, and the websites that you visited. If you are using our public

Wi-Fi network, we may, in addition, also collect the MAC address and name of your Wi-Fi device.

3. **Cookies.** A cookie is a small data file sent from your web browser to a web server and stored on your electronic device's hard drive. They are generated by websites to provide users with a personalized and often simplified online experience. You have the option of disabling such cookies if you choose not to allow their use. If you prefer, you can usually remove or reject browser cookies through the settings on your browser or device. Most web browsers are set to accept cookies by default. Keep in mind, though, that removing or rejecting cookies could affect the availability and functionality of our Library services.

You should be aware that information collected about you through any of the above means may be de-identified and aggregated with information collected about other users, visitors or donors. This de-identified and aggregated information cannot be used to reasonably identify you. This information helps us to administer services, analyze usage, provide security and identify new users of our Library services. In addition, it helps us to improve your user experience.

How does NYPL use the information collected?

Depending on the Library services you choose to use, the following are some examples of the ways we use your information in order to provide those services to you. You always have the option of whether or not to provide the information being used for such services.

- We use Personal Information and Residency Verification to issue Library cards. If a user chooses to provide an email address, NYPL may use it to send account alerts and other communications. We use Library Records to assist in maintaining our collections and to verify records of users' paid and unpaid fines.
- We use Shared Content, Login Credentials, Social Media Information and Library Records, as allowed by you and in accordance with the preferences you have established, to deliver enhanced or personalized services.
- We use Personal Information, Login Credentials, and Residency Verification to provide access to e-books through our mobile applications.
- We use Personal Information when collecting or processing payments, fines, and retail shop purchases.
- We use Personal Information and Social Media Information to administer promotions, surveys, and contests.
- We use Personal Information and Social Media Information to provide opportunities to further engage with the Library through advocacy and fundraising campaigns.

- We use cookies to collect information about your activity, browser, and device in order to provide you Library services. Cookies are used by us to remind us of who you are and help you navigate our website when you visit. Cookies also allow us to save your preferences so you do not have to reenter this information each time you use our Library services. You have the option of disabling cookies by using the settings on your web browser.

How do you manage information that NYPL has collected about you?

You can manage most information within your registered user account or you can ask our staff to assist you by phone at 1-917-ASK-NYPL, by emailing us at gethelp@nypl.org, or by visiting a Library location and speaking to our staff. Our information storage systems are configured in a way that helps us to protect information from accidental or malicious destruction. To that purpose, the information we collect is also saved in backup storage systems. Therefore, any update, change or deletion you make to your information or preferences may not immediately be reflected in all copies of the information we have and may not be removed from our backup storage systems until overwritten.

When does NYPL share information?

These are the ways NYPL shares your information with third-parties:

1. ***When You Share Content with the NYPL Community.*** If you choose to share content through our online services, the Shared Content may be publicly accessible. If you do not want to share content publicly, you can use your privacy settings to limit sharing. You may delete some content that you shared, but some interactive shared content may persist in association with your registered user account, even after your account is terminated. Therefore, you should keep this in mind when participating in shared content activity through our Library services.

2. ***Third-Party Library Services Providers.*** We use third-party library service providers and technologies to help deliver some of our services to you. If and when you choose to use such services, we may share your information with these third parties, but only as necessary for them to provide services to NYPL. We may also display links to third-party services or content. By following links, you may be providing information (including, but not limited to Personal Information) directly to a third party, to us, or to both. You acknowledge and agree that NYPL is not responsible for how those third parties collect or use your information. Third parties must either agree to adhere to strict confidentiality obligations in a way that is consistent with this Privacy Policy and the agreements we enter into with them or we require them to post their own privacy policy. We encourage you to review the privacy policies of every third-party website or service that you visit or use, including those third parties with whom you interact with through our Library services.

3. ***Fundraising and Marketing Outreach.*** As is customary in the non-profit world, we may send requests to support the Library to people who have expressed interest in the Library's programs or services. In order to ensure the most efficient use of our resources, we use third party vendors to make sure the contact information we have for our users is current and to determine which users are most likely to provide support. We do not rent or sell your Personal Information but we do share names and postal addresses with other nonprofit cultural organizations. Sharing this information with other reputable charitable organizations is the most cost effective way to find new users, share program offerings, and identify new donors. If you would prefer that your information not be shared with other organizations, please contact our Development Office by phone at 212-930-0653 or email to friends@nypl.org. We may also use information collected about you to work with third party marketing vendors to show you ads on third-party websites about Library services in which we think you may be interested. We may also use your information to improve our marketing outreach by working with third-party vendors to build models to identify and reach new users online based on them displaying similar online behavior to our existing users. You can easily opt-out of such use of your information by clicking the 'unsubscribe' link at the bottom of any marketing or communications e-mail you receive from us, or click here to request removal. If you would prefer that your information not be used for marketing purposes, please contact our Communications and Marketing Office by submitting this contact form, by phone at: 212-592-7700, or email to: comms@nypl.org

4. ***Legal Requests.*** Sometimes the law requires us to share your information, such as if we receive a valid subpoena, warrant, or court order. We may share your information if our careful review leads us to believe that the law, including state privacy law applicable to Library Records, requires us to do so.

5. ***Funders and Other Contributors.*** We are able to offer our users optional programs and services that we would not otherwise be able to provide without the generous support of funders and contributors. These funds are often dependent on NYPL complying with the reporting requirements of the funder or contributor. If you participate in these optional programs and services, your information may be included in these reports. When appropriate and practical, we will identify the name of funders and contributors associated with our programs and services and information we may share with them in the registration materials.

How does NYPL collect and share children's information?

The Children's Online Privacy Protection Act (COPPA) regulates online collection of information from children under the age of 13. If you are under the age of 13, you may not be allowed to use our online services without your parent's or guardian's permission, especially when your personal information may be collected. Parents and guardians of children under the age of 13 may view their children's Library Records.

Parents and guardians of children between the ages of 13 and 17 (inclusive) may also view their children's Library Records, but require their children's consent. We may partner with third-party services to provide educational content for children. Parents and guardians should review those services' privacy policies before permitting their children to use them. Parents and guardians may also need to sign additional consent forms for the collection of information about their children before they gain access to optional programs and services, such as our enrolled programs.

For more information

If you have questions or concerns about our Privacy Policy and practices, please send us an e-mail at: privacy@nypl.org

© The New York Public Library, 2017

SAMPLE FORM 6.2

The National Network of Libraries of Medicine (NNLM)

The Consumer Health Reference Interview and Ethical Issues

Finding quality health information is not always an easy process. Consumers often need assistance in locating appropriate resources to answer information requests. Librarians and library staff may face some important challenges during the health reference interview, the initial point of interaction between the consumer and the staff member. Consumers often consult other sources before coming to the library. For example, consumers may hear or read about health topics in the news, and they often discuss health concerns with family members or friends. They often search the Internet for health information and find varying degrees of quality. The library may actually be considered a "last resort" for some people searching for health information.

Note: When the term "librarian" appears below, the intended meaning includes all library staff members who provide reference and information services.

The Consumer Health Reference Interview
Consumer health questions present special challenges to the reference interview process:

- Consumers may have incomplete information about their health condition, or they are unfamiliar with medical terminology.
- The information needed may be about a sensitive health issue, such as a mental health or sexual health condition. Stigma about the health condition may prevent the consumer from even approaching a staff member.
- The health concerns may be serious, life-altering, or life-endangering. In addition, the patron may be nervous, embarrassed, upset, and emotional. Often the individual or their loved one has been newly diagnosed with a condition.

Consumers may have unreasonable expectations about the information available. For instance, they may want an easy-to-read source that clearly explains their unique medical condition. They might want a straightforward answer to a complex medical question so that they can make clear-cut decisions about their medical treatment. In reality, this kind of information may be difficult or impossible to find.

Consumers may be concerned about confidentiality, anonymity, and security, especially about personal health information transmitted electronically. They may have concerns about the confidentiality of information they send via e-mail or a website.

- Consumers may be confused about the role of the library staff. They might assume that the librarian can advise them on making health care decisions.

- Library staff may be afraid of providing the wrong answer to the health information question.
- Library staff may be concerned about providing negative information to the patron.

The following factors can affect success in the consumer health reference interview:

- Can the question be answered? If the consumer is looking for a "cure" for an incurable condition, it will be unrealistic and frustrating to try to answer the question.
- Did the patron ask the real question? Here, the librarian's skills at asking open-ended, neutral questions can reveal the true information needed.
- Did the librarian understand the actual question?
- Can the best resources be identified, and are they readily available?

Ethical Considerations
Consider the following guidelines for the consumer health reference interview. (Adapted from Healthnet: Connecticut Consumer Health Information Network)

1. **Provide a welcoming, safe environment.** Because of the personal, sensitive nature of health topics, consumers may be reluctant to approach the library staff member. Use welcoming behaviors like making eye contact, smiling, and greeting the patron. Provide a private area to discuss confidential topics. If there is not adequate privacy at the reference desk, take the person to the book stacks, an office, or another quiet area. Lower your voice if needed to maintain privacy, and assure the patron that confidentiality will be maintained. Do not discuss any reference interactions with other staff members, unless professional expertise is needed to answer the question.
2. **Be aware of the person asking the question, but don't make assumptions.** Do not assume that the person asking the question is the person who has the health condition. Parents, other family members, or friends may be asking for information for their loved one. Determine the age and sex of the person in question. A medical condition may affect a child differently than an adult, and treatments can vary depending on age and sex. Also, be aware of the person's emotional state. The patron may be upset and not clear about the information he or she needs. Keep your own emotions in check, and remain neutral. Be empathetic, patient, and non-judgmental. Be aware of your own body language.
3. **Get as much information as possible.** Use open-ended, neutral questions to find as much information as possible about what the person wants to know. If the individual is reluctant to divulge this information because of the nature of the health condition, share your reasons for wanting to know. Consider saying, "It will help me to find the information you need if you can tell me more about

what you want to know." You can save a great deal of time by determining what the person already knows about the subject. What sources has he or she already consulted? Were these sources too detailed, not detailed enough, too technical, or too general?

4. **Verify medical terminology in a medical dictionary or encyclopedia.** A consumer might not know the correct medical terminology to describe his or her health condition. Always verify unfamiliar terms in a dictionary or encyclopedia (both available in MedlinePlus). Be vigilant with medication names—some drugs have similar names but very different uses. Searching NLM's Drug Information Portal can be useful; start typing the drug name into the search box and suggested terms will begin to appear.

5. **Be aware of the limitations of medical information.** If appropriate, explain to the person the limitations of medical information, particularly that information becomes quickly outdated, that medical experts do not always agree about how to diagnose and treat a specific disease, and that most medical information is written in technical terms. Know when you have reached the limits of your collection, and explain these limitations to the consumer. This may include the fact that currency and scope limit any collection. Be prepared to send users to other valid sources of information.

6. **Provide the most complete information to answer the information request.** Providing the best, most accurate information is the goal of every reference interaction. This includes providing the most current and complete information possible and citing the source. However, some situations pose practical or ethical concerns. For example, some questions are far too broad to answer completely. A patron may ask for "everything you have about diabetes" or some other topic, in which the library staff will need to help the patron narrow down the question. For complex questions, the librarian can work with the patron to break it into manageable "chunks," providing information that can be digested a bit at a time. Offer to take the search to a higher level if the patron desires. Another challenge is that some library staff may feel uncomfortable or unwilling to provide an answer that is perceived to be bad news, such as a diagnosis that is debilitating or even fatal. However, such information should not be withheld; the role of the librarian is to provide the complete answer, not to censor out parts of the answer or to guess that the patron does not want the full answer. It is always appropriate to encourage the individual to discuss the issue with his or her health care provider instead of interpreting the information on their own, since every situation is unique.

7. **Do not interpret medical information or provide advice.** It is critical that you do not attempt to interpret medical information, provide a diagnosis, or recommend a therapy or intervention. Emphasize to your patron that you are an information professional, not a health professional. Avoid agreeing or disagreeing with what the consumer expresses. Do not offer your own experiences or hearsay about similar medical conditions. When discussing consumer

health issues in person, on the telephone, or via e-mail, state the limitations of your role as an information professional and the limitations of your collection. Advise the patron to consult with his or her health care provider for interpretation or explanation of the information. Add a disclaimer statement to library publications, including signage and e-mail signature blocks. Sample wording for disclaimers is available at the Disclaimers page on the Consumer and Patient Health Information Section (CAPHIS) website.

8. **Provide referrals.** Because library staff cannot provide medical advice, it is always good practice to refer the patron back to his or her health care professional to discuss the information they just received. It is also appropriate to provide access to directories or listings of health professionals and other organizations as needed. Use Health Hotlines (a directory of organizations with toll-free numbers) or MedlinePlus to access Directories and Organizations to find a local, state, or national organization dedicated to a specific health condition or concern. A referral as described is not the same as a recommendation. Do not provide recommendations to any health care service providers or organizations.

REFERENCES

ALA (American Library Association). n.d. "Questions and Answers on Privacy and Confidentiality." http://www.ala.org/advocacy/intfreedom/librarybill/interpretations/qu-privacy.

ALA (American Library Association). 2005. "Confidentiality and Coping with Law Enforcement Inquiries: Guidelines for the Library and Its Staff." April 2005. http://www.ala.org/Template.cfm?Section=ifissues&Template=/ContentManagement/ContentDisplay.cfm&ContentID=21654. Accessed March 7, 2017.

MLA (Medical Library Association). 2010. "Code of Ethics for Health Sciences Librarianship." June 2010. http://www.mlanet.org/p/cm/ld/fid=160.

New York Public Library. 2016. "New York Public Library Privacy Policy." November 30, 2016. https://www.nypl.org/help/about-nypl/legal-notices/privacy-policy.

NNLM (National Network of Libraries of Medicine). n.d. "The Consumer Health Reference Interview and Ethical Issues." https://nnlm.gov/professionaldevelopment/topics/ethics.

7

Community Outreach Planning

Takeaways from this chapter:

- *Outreach planning: step-by-step*
- *How to write a logic model*
- *How to measure program results*
- *Outreach programs*
- *Marketing strategies*

In business, as in life, it's generally a good idea to heed the old adage "Never assume anything," and certainly don't take anything (or anyone) for granted. Any library wanting to see its consumer health collection reach and be used by those for whom it is intended must be proactive, making every effort to reach out to prospective users. It's a dangerous idea for any library to simply assume that all (or even most) of the members of the community it serves even know about the library, think the library is the place to go for their health information needs, and know exactly what information can be found at the library. It's up to the library to make every possible effort to ensure that the community it serves is made aware of the treasure trove of information and programming available to them.

As discussed in chapters 1 and 2, it's imperative that any library have a detailed needs assessment of its community, including its demographics, environment, and, most importantly, its health issues and risks. As part of such fact-finding missions, community stakeholders, "those with a vested interest in the availability of health information resources" (Burroughs and Wood 2000, 6), have been identified and approached, with the goal of establishing a relationship and rapport for future shared projects. In libraries that are part of larger institutions, "champions" of outreach projects have been identified.

Now the all-important next step is to convene and collaborate with library staff, library stakeholders, and library champions to reach out to the library's community. First and foremost, outreach planners should decide the following:

- What exactly will the focus of the outreach program be? The library may be seeking to announce a new consumer health collection, ensure awareness of an existing consumer health collection, focus in on a specific health issue and risk of the community (e.g., diabetes, specific cancers in high numbers in that area), or alerting the community to high levels of lead in the drinking water.
- Who? Not only must the target audience be determined, but also the most effective partners in this mission must be identified.
- How will it be marketed or advertised and in what form? Print (e.g., flyers and posters), media (print, social, radio), or some combination of these?
- Where will it be marketed or advertised? Some examples are community civic or social organizations, faith-based organizations, schools and/or colleges, housing complexes, sports arenas or parks, supermarkets, and stores.

While libraries are, ultimately, businesses (or departments of businesses, e.g., hospitals, health centers, schools), there is a special element to them not found in other types of business. At its core, librarianship is a service profession; indeed, it can even be said that there is an altruistic element to the profession, as every librarian in every library setting is working to connect people with information, information that is their right to be able to access and understand. With regard to consumer health information, the New York State *Patients' Bill of Rights* includes, in part, the right to "participate in all decisions about your treatment and discharge" (NYS, n.d.) and the concept of "patient engagement," or ensuring that patients fully understand their case has been described as "the blockbuster drug of the century" (Dentzer 2013, 202).

What better way to serve patrons than by guiding them to an understanding of their health concerns and improving their health in some way. Patients and their loved ones are at an especially vulnerable point in their lives, and health literacy, simply stated the ability to understand and process health information, is a big problem. Now more than ever librarians must be proactive, and working with their community in an outreach project is a wonderful way to serve.

Armed with data, "in consultation with your team of advisors, determine if a project in your target community is needed and feasible" (Olney and Barnes 2013a, 2). Along with all the socioeconomic and demographic information gathering referred to in chapters 1 and 2 of this book, listening to stakeholders and partners will enable the library to decide on the project they want to tackle. And don't forget that special element—experienced librarians—who will have a strong sense of what is needed by their customers. Librarians new to the profession will bring not only the latest skill set, but also a fresh look at the project. And never forget to turn to the library's NNLM region for professional assistance, education, ideas, partnerships, and maybe even funding!

Outstanding resources for any library planning community outreach are the works of Cynthia A. Olney, currently acting assistant director of the National Network of Libraries of Medicine (NNLM) Outreach Evaluation Resource Center, and Susan J. Barnes.

Their three-part series, *Planning & Evaluating Health Information Outreach Projects,* now in a 2013 2nd edition, are available free and consist of Booklet One: *Getting Started with Community-Based Outreach,* Booklet Two: *Planning Outcomes-Based Outreach Projects,* and Booklet Three: *Collecting and Analyzing Evaluation Data.* In addition, all three are available online at the NNLM Evaluation Office (NEO) website.

Another great resource, also available free, is Catherine M. Burroughs and Fred B. Wood's 2000 work *Measuring the Difference: Guide to Planning and Evaluating Health Information Outreach.* In this case, the year of publication should not be a deterrence, as it offers useful and pertinent information. All four works present solid information with illustrative charts and sample planning forms, resources, references, and the all-important real-life examples of projects.

A good resource on partnerships is from the Urban Indian Health Institute (UIHI), a Division of the Seattle Indian Health Board, "Resource Guide I: Establishing and Maintaining Effective Partnerships" (UIHI 2011). UIHI makes an interesting point: "Members of a partnership may have a shared vision but that does not mean they have shared needs. . . . Differing agendas should be acknowledged so that they can be supported by the partnership." So if a college needs a formal publication as the result of a partnership, but the community member needs increased resources, there can still be a very effective partnership in the health program.

LOGIC MODEL

By now it should be clear that the all-important first step is a community assessment, which has been covered in prior chapters. The second step in an outreach project is creating a logic model. The logic model will help the library conceptualize the planned project in order to see how the project is meant to work and for what purpose. As Olney and Barnes emphasize, "In project planning, if you first identify your intended results, you are more likely to plan and conduct activities that will get you there. Also, you need to articulate your outcomes so you are sure to measure them and demonstrate to others the effectiveness of your project" (2013b, 1).

Olney (2017) states that "logic models just may be the duct tape of the evaluation world." Table 7.1 provides a "Logic Model Template" that can be used by all. She goes on to explain her "Logic Model 101," "Project Reality Check." She identifies "Reality Checkers" as stakeholders, experienced colleagues, and key informants. Olney suggests presenting these reality checkers with the library's one-page project vision, and ask them to assess it, and offers three questions for them to consider and answer:

- Are there resources in the community or in our partner organization that might help us do this project?

Table 7.1. Logic Model Template

Program: Health Information Outreach Program

Goal: Improve community members' abilities to find, evaluate, and use health information

Inputs	Activities		Outcomes		
			Why This Project: Short-Term Results	Why This Project: Intermediate Results	Why This Project: Long-Term Results
What We Invest	What We Do	Who We Reach	Learning	Action	Conditions
• Staff • Volunteers • Time • Money • Research findings • Materials • Equipment • Technology • Partners	• Conduct workshops and meetings • Train • Deliver services • Develop products, curricula, resources • Facilitate access to information • Work with media	• Participants • Clients • Agencies and community-based organizations (CBOs) • Decision-makers • Customers • Clinical professionals • Members of CBOs	• Awareness • Knowledge • Attitudes • Skills • Opinions • Aspirations • Motivations	• Behavior • Practice • Decision-making • Policies • Social Action	• Health • Social • Economic • Civic • Environmental

Assumptions
- Beliefs about the environment and community
- Should be confirmed before beginning the program

External Factors
- Positive and negative influences
- Culture, economics, politics, demographics
- Should be confirmed before beginning the program

Table 7.2. Logic Model Complete

Playbook: "Health Sciences Library Outreach on the Chicopee Public Library Bookmobile"

Goals:
1. Increase community awareness of consumer health information services provided by libraries.
2. Increase community access to reliable consumer health information services provided by libraries. Each partner materially invests in the program.

Inputs	Activities		Outcomes		
What We Invest	What We Do	Who We Reach	Why We Do It: Short-Term	Why We Do It: Intermediate	Why We Do It: Long-Term
HSL contributes pamphlets, Info Rx pads, large envelopes, bookmarks, business cards. HSL contributes librarian for scheduled visits, and to handle Info Rx requests. CPL contributes vehicle, Wi-Fi hot spot, librarian, CPL resources and services.	HSL selects and supplies pamphlets. HSL collects Info Rx/envelopes. HSL handles requests/mailings. HSL librarian makes scheduled visits to demo MedlinePlus on iPad. CPL librarian promotes and distributes pamphlets. CPL librarian handles requests as time permits.	Chicopee/Hampden County community members visiting: Boys and Girls Club City parks Councils on Aging Farmer's Market Federally funded housing complexes	Establish a baseline of CHI interactions through the number of iPad demonstrations and the number of Information Rx requests.	Measure community willingness to consider using libraries, including MedlinePlus, in meeting future CHI needs.	Measurable increase in community members reporting willingness to use library resources when facing medical decisions.

Assumptions:
HSL/CPL librarians will follow the procedures of the plan.
Community members will be interested in obtaining CHI from the Bookmobile.

External Factors:
(+) Participating in health fairs increases CHI requests.
(+) Bookmobile had a successful inaugural year.
(−) Unpredictability of community attendance at any outdoor event.
(−) Ebbs and flows of community interest in health topics.

Wood, Sandy, ed. *Consumer Health and Information Services and Programs: Best Practices.* Lanham, MD: Rowman & Littlefield, 2014, 97. Reprinted with permission from Rowman & Littlefield.

- Are there barriers or challenges we should be prepared to address?
- Please check the library project's team assumptions that they are making.

In addition, Olney (2016) offers the following advice: figure out what you're doing before you begin; in other words, begin with the end in mind. She gives the top five reasons for this approach:

- Outcomes are motivating.
- Outcomes help you focus.
- Outcomes provide a reality check.
- Planned outcomes set the final scene for your project story.
- Identifying expected outcomes helps you notice the unexpected.

Being able to measure your outcomes and demonstrate the effectiveness of your project is an excellent model to follow; it will be required if your project is funded by a grant, and offers solid information to present to administration, community stakeholders, and for future reference and examination.

So what does a logic model look like?

As it is always beneficial to see how models are implemented in a real-life situation, the completed logic model from the successful collaborative outreach between a hospital library (Baystate Health) and a public library (Chicopee Public Library) (Malachowski, Gancarz, and Brassil 2016) is shown in table 7.2.

COLLECTING AND ANALYZING EVALUATION DATA

As a good practice and as a mandatory element of grants, the outcomes of the outreach project, the data obtained, must be collected, analyzed, and reported.

While this may seem to some to be a daunting task, it need not be. In fact, this process should be looked at as a positive element of the program, as it can serve to show the program's success. In addition, it will be an opportunity for the library to demonstrate its value and its "return on investment."

Olney and Barnes describe this second step, process assessment, as a way to "track program progress, quality and lessons learned" (2013b, 9). This involves devising process questions, information to collect, and methods to do so (2013b, 10). In effect, the library is asking "So how'd we do?" in a formal, step-by-step manner. Process questions include:

- To what extent were you able to implement your project as planned?
- To what extent were you able to conduct specific activities as they were planned?
- How much community interest and activity did your project generate?
- To what extent did you reach your intended community?

- How effective were your recruitment strategies for attracting community members?
- What situational factors in the environment, community, or organizations affected project implementation?

To assist in process assessment, refer to Olney and Barnes's "Process Assessment Questions and Methods" (2013b, 23). Table 7.3 provides "Process Assessment Questions & Methods," and Table 7.4 provides "Objectives & Methods."

Examples of collecting information can run the gamut from tracking the number of participants or asking participants to fill out a straightforward Likert-style rating scale, to more complex feedback forms or even focus groups with participants. Recall the previously quoted words of Shipman and Lake, "If you've seen one consumer library, you have seen one consumer library" (Shipman and Lake 2014, 77). Every consumer library is unique unto itself, and every outreach project will be crafted to the needs of its community.

Don't forget the importance of the "human" element of assessing the project. All staff and shareholders involved should have "feedback sessions," and share "observations of activities" (Olney and Barnes 2013b, 10). Don't underestimate the importance of this, as often those in the thick of a project and those outside looking in will have different views of how well an event went. And don't overlook what may seem like trivial matters. Sometimes running out of an event "giveaway" can have some impact.

The next step is to evaluate data. "If you are going to make good decisions about your outreach project—or any other project—you need information or *data*" (Olney and Barnes 2013c, 1; author's italics). There are two methods to evaluate data, quantitative and qualitative. Simply put, any piece of information that can be counted is considered quantitative data, including:

- Attendance at classes or events
- Participation or drop-out rates
- Satisfaction ratings (Olney and Barnes 2013c, 2)

Some examples of commonly used quantitative methods include:

- End-of-session evaluations
- Tests (best if conducted before and after training, if applicable)
- Surveys
- Follow-up surveys (conducted some time period after)
- Attitude or opinion scales (e.g., Likert-type scale, strongly agree, agree)
- Dichotomous scales (yes/no) (Olney and Barnes 2013c, 3)

Qualitative methods, on the other hand, gather numerical data that is analyzed using statistical procedures and can provide rich details about the project (Olney and Barnes 2013c, 1).

Table 7.3. Worksheet Blank—Process Assessment Questions & Methods

Process Questions	Information to Collect	Methods
To what extent were you able to implement your project as planned?		
To what extent were you able to conduct specific activities as they were planned?		
How much community interest and activity did your project generate?		
To what extent did your reach your intended community?		
How effective were your recruitment strategies for attracting community members?		
What situational factors in the environment, community, or organizations affected project implementation?		

Table 7.4. Worksheet Blank—Objectives & Methods

Objective		
Measurable Indicator:		
Target:		
Time Frame:		
Data Source	Evaluation Method	Data Collection Timing

Objective		
Measurable Indicator:		
Target:		
Time Frame:		
Data Source	Evaluation Method	Data Collection Timing

Objective		
Measurable Indicator:		
Target:		
Time Frame:		
Data Source	Evaluation Method	Data Collection Timing

For those who are mathematically challenged, the two methods are clearly defined and illustrated. Information gathered must be coded, and then coded data must be organized and analyzed. Ideally, data should include both quantitative and qualitative.

Collecting and analyzing both types of data share four important steps:

- Design the data collection methods.
- Collect the data.
- Summarize and analyze the data.
- Access the validity of the findings. (Olney and Barnes 2013c, 38)

MARKETING

To paraphrase E. M. Forster in *Howards End*, "Only connect! The consumer and the health information!" As Davis asserts, "Marketing is the entire effort to connect the consumer with the product and keep the customer coming back for more" (2014, 187). So how does the library get its message out and what is the best way to do so?

Public libraries will more than likely already have a publicity or marketing department, or an individual assigned to this work. And for libraries that are part of larger institutions such as hospitals or universities, there will most definitely be a marketing department, which might also be called the department of communications or external affairs. Library staff involved in the consumer health community outreach program should arrange to meet with this department or specific employee to strategize the best way to market or publicize the program. This would include the best places to do so. A full understanding of the program, what it is, what it's looking to accomplish, and who it's meant to reach, should be clearly defined and discussed.

How the message gets out will depend entirely on the program and who it's targeting. The goal is to reach the target audience in the best way possible. For example, if the program is for teens, social media might be the best way to reach them, including email and tweets. All programs should appear on the library's Facebook page. Is the library working in conjunction with a community stakeholder? That individual would be the best source of advice on how to proceed. Eye-catching flyers can be distributed to, depending on the targeted audience, schools, community civic centers, organizations, workplaces, places of worship, and so forth, and should be not only in English but also in the language or languages of the targeted audiences.

No time to read through Olney and Barnes's work? The NNLM Evaluation Office (NEO) offers a four-step quick way to jump right in (https://nnlm.gov/neo/members/evaluationresources) as shown in Sample Form 7.1.

SAMPLE FORM 7.1

Four-Step Proposal Writing

4 Steps to an Evaluation Plan

Writing a proposal? Evaluation planning starts right when you start thinking about doing a project. We recommend working through the NEO's <u>Booklets,</u> but here are some of the basic steps and worksheets if you want to jump right in.

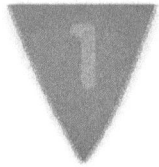

Do a Community Assessment

A community assessment helps you determine the health information needs of the community, the community resources that would support your project, and information to guide you in your choice and design of outreach strategies.

- Get organized
    - Network and identify a team of advisors
        - Suggested <u>networking opportunities</u>
        - <u>Book1 Worksheet: Networking</u>
    - Conduct a literature review
    - Take an inventory of what you already know and what you don't know (<u>SWOT Analysis</u>)
    - Develop <u>community assessment questions</u>
- Collect data about the community
    - Secondary sources (some <u>suggestions</u>)
    - Primary sources (interviews, focus groups, questionnaires, observations, site visits, online discussions)
        - <u>Book 1 Worksheet: Site Visit</u>
- <u>Interpret findings and make project decisions</u>

NEO Shop Talk Example <u>Assessing a Military Community</u>

Make a Logic Model

A logic model is a planning tool to clarify and graphically display how your activities are logically linked to the impact you hope to make with your project.

- How to do it (work from right to left, starting with outcomes)
- Outcomes are the results or benefits of your project - **Why** you are doing the project
    - short-term outcomes such as changes in knowledge
    - intermediate outcomes such as changes in behavior
    - long-term outcomes such as changes in individuals' health or medical access, social conditions or population health
- Logic Model Blank Worksheet Book 2 Worksheet: Logic Models
- Sample Logic Model

NEO Shop Talk Example Logic Model for a Birthday Party; Steering by Outcomes: Begin with the End in Mind

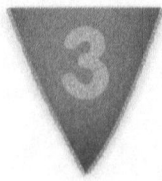

Develop Measurable Objectives for Your Outcomes

Outcomes are the results you are pursuing with your project. Measurable objectives communicate the evidence you will collect to show results and your criteria for determining success.

- For your outcomes (mostly short-term and intermediate), identify
    - Indicators (observable signs of the outcome)
    - Target criteria (level that must be attained to determine success)
    - Time frame (the point in time when the threshold for success will be achieved)
- How to do it

Community Outreach Planning 95

- Write your measurable objectives
    - Outcome Objective Blank Worksheet (the top section) Book 2 Worksheet: Outcome Objectives
    - Sample Outcome Objective using Success Criteria
    - Sample Outcome Objective using Change over Time

NEO Shop Talk Example Developing Program Outcomes Using the Kirkpatrick Model - With Vampires; Setting a Meaningful Participation Target

Create an Evaluation Plan

- Process Evaluation: Are you doing what you said you'd do?
    - Process Evaluation Blank Worksheet Book 2 Worksheet: Process Evaluation
    - Sample Process Evaluation Questions and Evaluation Methods
- Outcome Evaluation: Are you accomplishing the WHY of what you wanted to do?
    - Outcome Objective Blank Worksheet (the bottom section): Book 2 Worksheet: Outcome Objectives
        - Data Source: Examples of Data Sources
        - Evaluation Method: Examples of Evaluation Methods
        - Data Collection Timing: When you collect the data (ie. immediately after training, at the end of the project, etc.)

NEO Shop Talk Example The Kirkpatrick Model (Part 2) - With Humans

Librarians with consumer health collections should be on a proactive mission to get their much-needed information to their community. Of course, this might first involve alerting and educating members of the community that the collection exists and how it will benefit them. One of the best ways to do this is by reaching outside the library and connecting with community stakeholders and forging a firm partnership that will benefit all involved.

REFERENCES

Burroughs, Catherine M., and Fred B. Wood. 2000. *Measuring the Difference: Guide to Planning and Evaluating Health Information Outreach.* Seattle, WA: National Network of Libraries of Medicine, Pacific Northwest Region.

Davis, Jackie. 2014. "Marketing Health Library Services to Patients and Consumers." In *The Medical Library Association Guide to Providing Consumer and Patient Health Information*, edited by Michele Spatz, 185–98. Lanham, MD: Rowman & Littlefield.

Dentzer, Susan. 2013. "Rx for the 'Blockbuster Drug' of Patient Engagement." *Health Affairs* 32, no. 2: 202.

Malachowski, Margot, Anne Gancarz, and Ellen Brassil. 2016. "Collaborative Outreach between a Hospital Library and a Public Library." In *Consumer Health Information Services and Programs: Best Practices*, edited by M. Sandra Wood, 87–101. Lanham, MD: Rowman & Littlefield.

NYS (New York State). n.d. *Patients' Bill of Rights.* Public Health Law (PHL) 2803 (1)(g) Patients' Rights, 10NYCRR, 405.7, 405.7 (a) (1), 405.7 (c).

Olney, Cindy. 2016. "Steering by Outcomes: Begin with the End in Mind." NNLM NEO news. May 20, 2016. https://news.nnlm.gov/neo/2016/05/20/steering-by-outcomes-begin-with-the-end-in-mind/.

Olney, Cindy. 2017. "A Logic Model Hack: The Project Reality Check." NNLM. *NEO Shop Talk* (blog). February 24, 2017. https://news.nnlm.gov/neo/2017/02/24/a-logic-model-hack-the-project-reality-check/.

Olney, Cynthia A., and Susan J. Barnes. 2013a. *Getting Started with Community-Based Outreach.* 2nd ed. *Planning and Evaluating Health Information Outreach Projects Booklet One.* Seattle, WA: National Network of Libraries of Medicine, Pacific Northwest Region. https://nnlm.gov/neo/guides/bookletOne508.

Olney, Cynthia A., and Susan J. Barnes. 2013b. *Planning Outcomes-Based Outreach Projects.* 2nd ed. *Planning and Evaluating Health Information Outreach Projects Booklet Two.* Seattle, WA: National Network of Libraries of Medicine, Pacific Northwest Region. https://nnlm.gov/neo/guides/bookletTwo508.

Olney, Cynthia A., and Susan J. Barnes. 2013c. *Collecting and Analyzing Evaluation Data.* 2nd ed. *Planning and Evaluating Health Information Outreach Projects Booklet Three.* Seattle, WA: National Network of Libraries of Medicine, Pacific Northwest Region. https://nnlm.gov/neo/guides/bookletThree508.

Shipman, Jean, and Erica Lake. 2014. "Prized Assets: Staff." In *The Medical Library Association Guide to Providing Consumer and Patient Health Information*, edited by Michele Spatz, 77–95. Lanham, MD: Rowman & Littlefield.

Urban Indian Health Institute. Seattle Indian Health Board. 2011. *Resource Guide I: Establishing and Maintaining Effective Partnerships.* http://www.uihi.org/download/Resource-Guide-1-Establishing-and-Maintaing-Effective-Partnerships.pdf.

8

Health Literacy and Librarians

Takeaways from this chapter:

- *What health literacy is*
- *How librarians can help*
- *How it affects choice of consumer health materials*

Why a chapter on health literacy? And what is health literacy anyway? And what do librarians have to do with this? Librarians with a consumer health collection need to be aware of and fully understand the importance of the concept and be able to choose materials for their collection that address the issue. If patrons cannot fully understand the materials given to them by their librarian, the information is useless. Yes, of course, it's not really up to the librarian to "test" each patron to determine his or her level of health literacy, but by being aware of this pervasive problem, librarians can keep this issue in mind when dispensing information, just as they are mindful of providing materials in languages other than English, and in large print.

So what exactly is meant by the term "health literacy"?

While there are several definitions of health literacy, this chapter will make use of the definition developed for the National Library of Medicine and used by Healthy People 2020: "The degree to which individuals have the capacity to obtain, process, and understand basic health information and services needed to make appropriate health decisions" (1).

NNLM's excellent overview of the subject on their website (https:nnlm.gov/professional-development/topics/health-literacy) explains the skills needed for health literacy that underscore the complexity of this issue:

Skills Needed for Health Literacy

Patients are often faced with complex information and treatment decisions. Patients need to:

- Access health care services
- Analyze relative risks and benefits
- Calculate dosages
- Communicate with health care providers
- Evaluate information for credibility and quality
- Interpret test results
- Locate health information

In order to accomplish these tasks, individuals may need to be:

- Visually literate (able to understand graphs or other visual information)
- Computer literate (able to operate a computer)
- Information literate (able to obtain and apply relevant information)
- Numerically or computationally literate (able to calculate or reason numerically)

Oral language skills are important as well. Patients need to articulate their health concerns and describe their symptoms accurately. They need to ask pertinent questions, and they need to understand spoken medical advice or treatment directions. In an age of shared responsibility between physician and patient for health care, patients need strong decision-making skills. With the development of the Internet as a source of health information, health literacy may also include the ability to search the Internet and evaluate Web sites.

The ability to navigate the increasingly complex health-care system with its short patient-provider interaction combined with the necessity for patients to become their own health advocate, or find a family member or friend who can fill this role for them, is daunting for anyone. To some it might seem commonsense to question or challenge their clinician, to seek second (or third) opinions, or read up on everything patients can get their hands on, but there are factors involved when it comes to health-care information that complicate or even prohibit these actions. Patrons may have limited education and limited reading abilities, and limited (or no) proficiency in English. Add to this the vulnerability of the consumer seeking health information, who is sick, scared, intimidated, overwhelmed, or any combination thereof.

Imagine not being able to read and understand the patient education material your health-care provider gives you. Or imagine thinking that if test results are "positive" it's a good thing. Or to not understand the instructions on the medications your clinician gave you. Why doesn't the consumer simply ask the doctor or the pharmacist? There can be a myriad of reasons. Consumers may be embarrassed, or maybe they feel that they do understand the material even though in reality they've misinterpreted it.

Just how much of a problem is health literacy? Unfortunately it's a big problem. The only national report offering data on the health literacy skills of Americans was published in 2006 by the US Department of Education. *The Health Literacy of America's Adults: Results from the 2003 National Assessment of Adult Literacy* (NAAL) reveals the astonishingly awful news that "the majority of adults (53 percent) had *Intermediate* health literacy. An additional 12 percent of adults had *Proficient* health literacy. Among the remaining adults, 22 percent had *Basic* health literacy, and 14 percent had *Below Basic* health literacy" (US Department of Education 2006, v; italics in original). The NAAL defines these categories as follows:

- *Below Basic* indicates no more than the most simple and concrete literacy skills.
- *Basic* indicates skills necessary to perform simple and everyday literacy activities.
- *Intermediate* indicates skills necessary to perform moderately challenging literacy activities.
- *Proficient* indicates skills necessary to perform more complex and challenging literacy activities.

And, of course, the health sciences field has its own "language," terminology, or jargon that only clinicians fully understand.

In March 2016 the US Department of Education released *Skills of U.S. Unemployed, Young, and Older Adults in Sharper Focus: Results from the Program for the International Assessment of Adult Competencies (PIAAC) 2012/2014: First Look*. The study charted adults' proficiencies in three areas: literacy, numeracy, and problem solving in technology-rich environments. Proficiencies levels ranged from "below level 1," the lowest, to "level 5," the highest.

The "overall summary for U.S. adults age 16–65 by employment status" showed that only "15 percent of employed adults age 16–65 performed at the top proficiency level"; in numeracy "12 percent of employed adults reached this level" (US Department of Education 2016, 5).

And let's not forget that, as mentioned in chapter 1, according to the Pew Research Center (2013), despite these limitations, 72 percent of Americans say they sought health information online in the past year, and 77 percent of online health seekers say they began with a search engine.

Fortunately, the health-care system is very much aware of this issue and increasingly makes efforts to alleviate it. In fact, the Agency for Healthcare Research and Quality (AHRQ), part of the US Department of Health and Human Services, issued the "AHRQ Health Literacy Universal Precautions Toolkit" in 2010, with a second edition in 2015. AHRQ's recommendation to clinicians is to assume that *everyone* may have difficulty relating their health issues and understanding the information their clinician provides. While we tend to assume that only poorly educated or underserved populations will have problems with health literacy, it is not impossible for even highly educated individuals to not fully comprehend their health-care experience. It cannot be overstated how exhausting and daunting dealing with the health-care system is, so *everyone* needs special attention at this time of stress and psychological and emotional vulnerability.

So what part do librarians play in this? Several points of both the American Library Association's "Core Values of Librarianship" http://www.ala.org/advocacy/intfreedom/corevalues), and its "Code of Ethics of the American Library Association" (http://www.ala.org/tools/ethics) and the Medical Library Association's "Code of Ethics for Health Sciences Librarianship: Goals and Principles for Ethical Conduct" (http://www.mlanet.org/page/code-of-ethics) are particularly pertinent to this issue. MLA avers that "the health sciences librarian believes that knowledge is the *sine qua non* of informed decisions in health care" and its statements include "The health sciences librarian promotes access to health information for all and creates and maintains conditions of freedom, inquiry, thought, and expression that facilitate informed health care decisions," and "The health sciences librarian ensures that the best available information is provided to the client." ALA, in its "Core Values of Librarianship," states that "all information resources that are provided directly or indirectly by the library, regardless of technology, format, or methods of delivery, should be readily, equally, and equitably accessible to all library users," and the "Code of Ethics of the American Library Association" states in Article I that "we provide the highest level of service to all library users through appropriate and usefully organized resources; equitable service policies; equitable access; and accurate, unbiased, and courteous responses to all requests." As Jeffrey T. Davis so well puts it, "Reducing barriers to access is a library value" (2017, 94). And certainly, providing patrons with understandable health-care information that will enable them to make informed decisions is downright destroying one huge barrier.

Librarians will most likely never be called upon to actually write health-related material, or if they do it would most likely be in partnership with a clinician partner; but they may, however, be assigned to write up publicity flyers or announcements for their customers regarding available resources or programming on health information, so it's wise for librarians to be aware of tools used to determine the level of difficulty of reading material, be it in print or online.

The National Library of Medicine's National Information Center on Health Services Research and Health Care Technology's (NICHSR) Health Services Research Information Council (HSRIC) offers an outstanding list of resources on "Health Literacy and Cultural Competence" (https://www.nlm.nih.gov/hsrinfo/health_literacy.html). These are the areas covered:

- Search Queries Using NLM and DHHS Resources: Health Literacy and Cultural Competency

- News: Health Literacy and Cultural Competence
- Data, Tools, and Statistics: Measurement Tools
- Guidelines, Journals, Other Publications
- Education
- Meetings/Conferences/Webinars: Past Meetings | Upcoming Meetings
- Key Organizations

Some tools to determine the reading level of materials include:

- SMOG (Simplified Measure of Gobbledygoop), first developed by G. Harry McLaughlin ("SMOG Grading—a New Readability Formula," *Journal of Reading* 12, no. 8 [1969]: 639–46); test available from University of South Carolina. Arnold School of Public Health
- Fry's Readability Graph available from Discovery School's Kathy Schrock's Guide for Educators (http://www.schrockguide.net/uploads/3/9/2/2/392267/fry_directions.pdf)
- The Agency for Healthcare Research and Quality (AHRQ) Health Literacy Measurement Tools (Revised) (https://www.ahrq.gov/professionals/quality-patient-safety/quality-resources/tools/literacy/index.html), includes the *Short Assessment of Health Literacy—Spanish and English*; *Rapid Estimate of Adult Literacy in Medicine—Short Form*; and *Short Assessment of Health Literacy for Spanish Adults*

While this is meant for clinicians, it is still of interest and value to all.

PLAIN LANGUAGE

There are numerous guides to writing "plain language" information for consumers. They include "Plain Language Materials & Resources," from the CDC (https://www.cdc.gov/healthliteracy/developmaterials/plainlanguage.html), which includes "Everyday Words for Public Health Communication"; this can be used by "anyone writing for an audience that will benefit from jargon-free language: Consider the intended audience, and use the language that will make the most sense to them. When you do need to reach a broad, public audience without specialized knowledge about a topic, everyday words are the most appropriate language to help the most people understand the information" (CDC 2016).

Another good resource is "Research-Based Health Literacy Materials and Instruction Guide: Beginning and Intermediate ABE and ESL Levels" from the Literacy Information and Communication System (https://lincs.ed.gov/health/health).

In addition, the National Library of Medicine's MedlinePlus section on "Easy-to-Read Materials" (MedlinePlus 2018) offers easy-to-read health information on a number of topics, most in English and Spanish, and includes a section on "How to Write Easy to Read Materials."

As mentioned in chapter 6, the National Network of Libraries of Medicine (NNLM) (https://nnlm.gov/) offers courses on consumer health information that are free and offered online and, for the most part, asynchronously. These courses can lead to Medical Library Association Consumer Health Information Specialization (CHIS) certification, both Level I and Level II. They offer a wealth of information and resources on consumer health. For example, one course, "The Canny Consumer: Resources for Consumer Health Decision-Making," includes lists of resources on "Talking to Your Doctor," "Getting a Copy of Your Medical Records," "Wellness and Nutrition," and "Informed Health Care Decisions." The latter includes such sites as PubMed Health (http:www.ncbi.nlm.nih.gov/pubmed-health), which provides information for consumers and clinicians on prevention and treatment of diseases and conditions. PubMed Health specializes in reviews of clinical effectiveness research, with easy-to-read summaries for consumers as well as full technical reports.

The CDC has a great resource, "Health Literacy Activities by State" (https://www.cdc.gov/healthliteracy/statedata/). Listed are the initiatives of nineteen states that are in line with the "National Action Plan to Improve Health Literacy" of the US Department of Health and Human Services, Office of Disease Prevention and Health Promotion (http://www.health.gov/communication/hlactionplan/pdf/Health_Literacy_Action_Plan.pdf).

The Institute for Healthcare Advancement (IHA) (http://www.iha4health.org) is a not-for profit organization "dedicated to empowering people to better health." Along with offering fee-based health literacy training and consulting services and organizing an annual continuing education health literacy conference, they publish and sell a variety of easy-to-read books in several languages.

HOW LIBRARIANS ARE HELPING TO IMPROVE HEALTH LITERACY IN THEIR COMMUNITIES: SOME PROGRAMS AND SOME IDEAS

All librarians are committed to serving their patrons and providing them with the best possible materials. But more than ever before it's become necessary to be proactive and reach out the library's patrons. Don't wait for them to come to the library; go to them. Since the advent of the internet, for better or worse, many are of a mind-set that they can easily find any information or all they may need by "googling" or turning to Facebook and other social media. Yet on the other hand, there is also a significant part of communities who simply do not know how to find any information, and who may be unaware of their library or unable to use it for various reasons.

Armed with their library's community assessments, and working with stakeholders and community organizations, librarians can create outreach programs to educate their patrons. And create they do! The outreach initiatives created by libraries and partners are remarkable.

Engage for Health: A Partnership for Improved Patient-Doctor Communication

The Hospital and Healthsystem Association of Pennsylvania (HAP) (https://haponline.org) is a nonprofit organization with more than 240 hospitals and health system members across the continuum of care. Their *HAP 2014–2016 Strategic Plan: Working to Achieve a Healthy Pennsylvania* (https://haponline.org/Portals/0/docs/About/2014-2016-HAP-Strategic-Plan.pdf) outlined their goals to focus on community health and well-being and improve the health of Pennsylvanians.

HAP and its Pennsylvania Hospital Engagement Network, PA-HEN (https://hapoline.org/quality), developed "Engage for Health," a "patient communication program," and launched it in October 2014, during Health Literacy Month. This program will enable and encourage community members to take an active role in their health care by preparing consumers for their encounters with their clinicians, educating them on how to be prepared and focus on questions that will aid them in decision-making.

In 2016, the Pennsylvania Library Association (www.palibraries.org) and the National Network of Libraries of Medicine, Middle Atlantic Region (NNLM MAR) (https://nnlm.gov/mar) partnered with HAP, the NNLM Evaluation Office (NEO) (https://nnlm.gov/neo), and the US Department of Health & Human Services Agency for Healthcare Research and Quality (AHRQ) (https://www.ahrq.gov) to update the program and pilot it in sixteen libraries across Pennsylvania.

Those sixteen libraries were trained on NNLM resources, evaluation techniques, and assisted in the creation of an evaluation tool specifically designed for the "Engage for Health" program. Those libraries were then able to offer the program in their community.

The "Engage for Health" program is now available for libraries, community and faith-based agencies and health-care providers. NNLM MAR has a site dedicated to this (https://nnlm.gov/mar/guides/engageforhealth) and offers a toolkit of free materials to present this program, including presentation slides and speaker notes; a role-play exercise; pre- and postevaluation forms; and promotional posters and logo. At the home page there is a video of the program that was hosted by the Hershey Public Library in Hershey, Pennsylvania.

In the pilot project, 150 adults participated; 132 completed evaluation forms. Ninety-eight percent rated the program positively. Interestingly, 92 percent had never used MedlinePlus, and 78 percent had never *heard* of MedlinePlus (EngageforHealth 2017)!

Focused Health Information Project

After identifying geographic areas that are medically underserved or economically disadvantaged, NNLM New England Region (NER) (https://nnlm.gov/ner) created the "Focused Health Information Outreach" initiative (https://nnlm.gov/ner/about/initiatives/focused-outreach), a five-year project that each year focused on two geographic areas, one rural and one urban. The project sought to connect with community-based organizations and other agencies in the targeted population.

The pilot year covered Providence, Rhode Island, and the Western Maine Health District; Year 1 covered Downeast District, Maine, and Holyoke, Massachusetts; Year 2 Northern Worcester County (Massachusetts) and Hartford, Connecticut; Year 3 Vermont; and Year 4, New Hampshire. Final reports of each year are available on the website cited above.

Year 4's initiative included several partners, including the New Hampshire State Library. A "train the trainer" approach was used, wherein librarians from each of New Hampshire's eleven library cooperatives were given instruction on how to use MedlinePlus.

Trained librarians in turn presented the same training at their cooperatives' meetings. Trainers were required to teach MedlinePlus, to encourage librarians in their cooperative to join the NNLM NER, and to add a link to MedlinePlus to their respective library's website. As a result of this project, 120 librarians were trained, twenty-nine libraries joined the NNLM NER, and forty-eight libraries added a link to MedlinePlus on their website (NNLM/NCR Focused Outreach).

Just for the Health of It

Since 2009, the East Brunswick (NJ) Public Library (EBPL), which serves a community of approximately forty-eight thousand residents, has been running "Just for the Health of It," a health literacy initiative to "deliver equal access trustworthy health and wellness information."

A $15,000 award from NNLM Middle Atlantic Region (MAR) enabled the library to improve its portal; in 2014 EBPL received two additional awards from MAR, $10,000 to redesign the health portal and $5,000 to market the newly redesigned health portal to the community. The portal includes links to authoritative and reliable consumer health websites; information about health workshops in area hospitals or at the library; a "health insurance marketplace calculator," articles, and videos. "Just for the Health of It" was recognized on January 20, 2017, by the New Jersey Hospital Association's "Outside the Box: Partnering with Local Libraries to Increase Community Health Literacy" (East Brunswick 2017).

These are just three examples of library health literacy outreach initiatives around the US. They serve to underscore not only the dedication and creativity of libraries, but also the positive results gained from partnerships with other community organizations.

SOME IDEAS FOR HEALTH LITERACY OUTREACH

Ideally, there should be health literacy components/lessons in all English as a second language (ESL) classes. Some programs are already in place. This could be an outstanding outreach program for libraries in partnership with literacy organizations, state and local government health agencies, and universities.

It should be noted for all the examples shown of health literacy components of ESL classes that while nearly all curriculums for both instructors and students are readily available for download on the internet, most come with some rules for use; these must be carefully and strictly followed. It should also be noted that any curriculums should be carefully reviewed to be sure they are suitable for the intended audience.

Florida Health Literacy Coalition "Staying Healthy for Beginners"

Staying Healthy (http://www.floridaliteracy.org/health_literacy_curriculum.html) is an award-winning curriculum that is used throughout the US. It is written at a fourth- to fifth-grade reading level and is suitable for low- to intermediate-level ESL learners and above. The newly released Staying Healthy for Beginners is written at a lower reading level, making it more accessible to learners at the high beginning level.

Lessons, teacher's guide, and other materials are available free for download. Some items are also available in print form; they're free for Florida literacy groups, but at a nominal charge for those outside of Florida.

Queens Library English for Your Health

Queens, New York, is one of the five boroughs of New York City. The Queens Library system serves 2.3 million people at sixty-two locations, including seven Adult Learning Centers and two Family Literacy Centers.

They have developed an "English for Your Health" program, developed for adults who speak very little English to learn about health topics (http://www.queenslibrary.org/services/health-info/english-for-your-health). The website includes online activities for students to try, and teacher lesson plans, student worksheets, and audio files for both beginner and intermediate levels. In addition, classes are taught at the library.

Library Information and Communication System (LINCS) "Research-Based Health Literacy Materials and Instruction Guide: Beginning and Intermediate ABE and ESL Levels"

LINCS, an initiative of the US Department of Education, Office of Career, Technical, and Adult Education (OCTAE), developed these health literacy materials to meet both the need of adults to enhance their literacy skills as well as their need to navigate the health-care system and begin to achieve better health care for themselves and their families. These materials integrate literacy skills and practice with pertinent health information. In a scientifically based research environment, use of these materials led to an increase in participants' literacy scores on standardized tests used to validate literacy gains. And, equally as important for these adult learners, they significantly increased health literacy and knowledge.

The materials presented at this site are specifically intended for beginning ABE (Adult Basic Education) and ESL (English as a Second Language) learners, and the strategies they employ to develop and strengthen the components of the reading process are those proven effective with these groups.

Expecting the Best

The Center for Literacy Studies at the University of Tennessee has developed "Expecting the Best," an ESL health and wellness curriculum. Student lessons and an instructor's manual are available for download (http://www.cls.utk.edu/expect thebest.html).

These programs are examples of health literacy instruction librarians may wish to consider for their libraries in partnership with local organizations, including hospitals and civic and faith-based groups.

KEEPING UP WITH HEALTH LITERACY

Along with involvement with the library's regional NNLM, librarians should subscribe to the e-newsletter of Helen Osborne, a recognized expert in the field of health literacy and president of Health Literacy Consulting. She founded Health Literacy Month (October), a worldwide campaign to raise awareness of this vital issue. Along with her e-newsletter, she offers free access to her podcast *Health Literacy Out Loud*, where she interviews experts on various aspects of health literacy (http://healthlit eracy.com).

Health literacy is a problem that affects many members of the community. Each library needs to ascertain the best way possible to reach out and help its patrons improve their health literacy with programs alone or in partnership with community stakeholders. The library's community's health literacy issues should be kept in mind when purchasing consumer health materials.

REFERENCES

American Library Association Code of Ethics. 2008. http://www.ala.org/tools/ethics.
American Library Association "Core Values of Librarianship." 2006. http://www.ala.org/ad vocacy/intfreedom/corevalues.

CDC Centers for Disease Control. 2016. *Plain Language Materials & Resources*. https://www.cdc.gov/healthliteracy/developmaterials/plainlanguage.html.

Davis, Jeffrey T. 2017. *The Collection All Around: Sharing Our Cities, Towns, and Natural Places*. Chicago: ALA.

East Brunswick, NJ *Public Library. Just for the Health of It!* Site. "Just for the Health of It was recognized by the New Jersey Hospital Association, January 20, 2017. http://www.wellinks.org/content/just-health-it-was-recognized-new-jersey-hospital-association.

LINCS Library Information and Communication System. U.S. Department of Education, Office of Career, Technical, and Adult Education (OCTAE). 2009. *Research-based Health Literacy Materials and Instruction Guide—Beginning and Intermediate ABE and ESL Levels*. https://lincs.ed.gov/health/health.

Medical Library Association, "Code of Ethics for Health Sciences Librarianship." 2010. http://www.mlanet.org/page/code-of-ethics.

MedlinePlus. National Institutes of Health / U.S. National Library of Medicine. 2018. *Easy-to-Read*. https://medlineplus.gov/all_easytoread.html.

National Network of Libraries of Medicine / Middle Atlantic Region NNLM/MAR Engage for Health Collaboration. 2017. *Findings from the Engage for Health Pilot Project*. https://nnlm.gov/sites/default/files/mar/files/1_PaLA_EngageforHealth_PilotProjectFindings UPDATE.pdf.

National Network of Libraries of Medicine / New England Region NNLM/NER. *Focused Health Information Outreach*. https://nnlm.gov/ner/about/initiatives/focused-outreach.

NNLM Health Literacy. n.d. https://nnlm.gov/priorities/topics/health-literacy.

Pew Research Center. 2013. *Pew Internet Health Online 2013*. http://www.pewinternet.org/files/old-media/Files/Reports/PIP_HealthOnline.pdf.

US Department of Education. 2006. *The Health Literacy of America's Adults: Results from the 2003 National Assessment of Adult Literacy*. http://nces.ed.gov/pubsearch/pubsinfo.asp?pubid=2006483.

US Department of Education. 2016. *Skills of U.S. Unemployed, Young, and Older Adults in Sharper Focus: Results from the Program for the International Assessment of Adult Competencies (PIAAC) 2012/2014: First Look*. March 2016. https://nces.ed.gov/pubs2016/2016039rev.pdf.

9
Multicultural/Inclusive Consumer Health Information

Takeaways from this chapter:

- *How to find best consumer health information and meet the needs of ALL patrons including multicultural, multilingual, and the LGBTQ communities*
- *How to create inviting and nonjudgmental inclusive environments*

Health information, like health care, is not "one size fits all." Librarians must be aware of the wide variety of health information that is available for all members of their communities. The consumer health collection should not only include information on women's health, men's health, and the health issues of different age groups, including infants, children, teens, adults, and seniors, but also information on how health issues may affect immigrant, ethnic, and racial groups differently. For example, some diseases are more prevalent in certain racial groups. According to the American Heart Association (2017), "The prevalence of high blood pressure in African-Americans is the highest in the world," and some health issues affect certain groups disproportionately due to educational, cultural, and socioeconomic reasons. According to the US Department of Health and Human Services' Indian Health Service (2017), "The American Indian and Alaska Native people have long experienced lower health status when compared with other Americans. Lower life expectancy and the disproportionate disease burden exist perhaps because of inadequate education, disproportionate poverty, discrimination in the delivery of health services, and cultural differences. These are broad quality of life issues rooted in economic adversity and poor social conditions." And, of course, these issues apply to any disadvantaged and underserved population.

Any consumer health collection must also include information for the community's LGBTQ population. "LGBTQ" (lesbian, gay, bisexual, transgender/transsexual, queer/questioning) is an umbrella term, but each group is unique and has their own unique health concerns.

The bottom line is that each library needs to create an inviting atmosphere for all members of its community. Every patron should be met in an open and friendly way, and their questions answered nonjudgmentally. As discussed in chapter 5, sensitivity training might be a good idea for staff. And, of course, this welcoming atmosphere needs to extend to the library's "internal customers," namely, staff members.

IMMIGRANT POPULATIONS

Part of any community assessment will include determining which immigrant populations are most prevalent in a library's community. There's no need to stock up on Spanish materials if the largest part of the immigrant population is from Vietnam. Of course, librarians must know how to find health information in a multitude of languages.

The Migration Policy Institute offers "State Immigration Data Profiles" (http://www.migrationpolicy.org/programs/data-hub/state-immigration-data-profiles) that give statistics on the number of immigrants and their countries of origin. And their "Migration Data Hub" (http://www.migrationpolicy.org/programs/migration-data-hub) "showcases the most current national and state-level demographic, social, and economic facts about immigrants to the United States," including unauthorized immigrants. And the US Census Bureau's American Fact Finder: Community Facts (https://factfinder.census.gov/faces/nav/jsf/pages/community_facts.xhtml) allows the user to search for information by zip code.

According to the Pew Research Center (2016), "Just 10 states resettled more than half of recent refugees," the top three being California, Texas, and New York. Across the United States there will be widely varying immigrant populations, including seasonal migrant workers.

The International Federation of Library Associations and Institutions (IFLA) and the United Nations Educational, Scientific and Cultural Organization (UNESCO) have written a Multicultural Library Manifesto (IFLA/UNESCO 2012). This is available in multiple languages. (See Sample Form 9.1.)

SAMPLE FORM 9.1

IFLA/UNESCO Multicultural Library Manifesto

The Multicultural Library—A Gateway to a Cultural Diverse Society in Dialogue

All people live in an increasingly heterogeneous society. There are more than 6,000 different languages in the world. The international migration rate is growing every year resulting in an increasing number of people with complex identities. Globalization, increased migration, faster communication, ease of transportation and other 21st century forces have increased cultural diversity in many nations where it might not have previously existed or has augmented the existing multicultural makeup.

"Cultural Diversity" or "Multiculturalism" refers to the harmonious co-existence and interaction of different cultures, where "culture should be regarded as the set of distinctive spiritual, material, intellectual and emotional features of society or a social group, and that it encompasses, in addition to art and literature; lifestyles, ways of living together, value systems, traditions and beliefs."[1] Cultural diversity or multiculturalism is the foundation of our collective strength in our local communities and in our global society.

Cultural and linguistic diversity is the common heritage of humankind and should be cherished and preserved for the benefit of all. It is a source for the exchange, innovation, creativity, and peaceful coexistence among peoples. "Respect for the diversity of cultures, tolerance, dialogue and cooperation, in a climate of mutual trust and understanding are among the best guarantees of international peace and security."[2] Therefore, libraries of all types should reflect, support and promote cultural and linguistic diversity at the international, national, and local levels, and thus work for cross-cultural dialogue and active citizenship.

As libraries serve diverse interests and communities, they function as learning, cultural, and information centres. In addressing cultural and linguistic diversity, library services are driven by their commitment to the principles of fundamental freedoms and equity of access to information and knowledge for all, in the respect of cultural identity and values.

---

[1] UNESCO Universal Declaration on Cultural Diversity, 2001.   [2] ibid

Principles

Each individual in our global society has the right to a full range of library and information services. In addressing cultural and linguistic diversity, libraries should:

- serve all members of the community without discrimination based on cultural and linguistic heritage;
- provide information in appropriate languages and scripts;
- give access to a broad range of materials and services reflecting all communities and needs;
- employ staff to reflect the diversity of the community, who are trained to work with and serve diverse communities.

Library and information services in a culturally and linguistically diverse context include both the provision of services to all types of library users and the provision of library services specifically targeted to underserved cultural and linguistic groups. Special attention should be paid to groups which are often marginalized in culturally diverse societies: minorities, asylum seekers and refugees, residents with a temporary residence permit, migrant workers, and indigenous communities.

Missions of Multicultural Library Services

In a culturally diverse society focus should be on the following key missions, which relate to information literacy, education and culture:

- promoting awareness of the positive value of cultural diversity and fostering cultural dialogue;
- encouraging linguistic diversity and respect for the mother tongue;
- facilitating the harmonious coexistence of several languages, including learning of several languages from an early age;
- safeguarding linguistic and cultural heritage and giving support to expression, creation and dissemination in all relevant languages;
- supporting the preservation of oral tradition and intangible cultural heritage;
- supporting inclusion and participation of persons and groups from all diverse cultural grounds;
- encouraging information literacy in the digital age, and the mastering of information and communication technologies;
- promoting linguistic diversity in cyberspace;
- encouraging universal access to cyberspace; supporting the exchange of knowledge and best practices with regard to cultural pluralism.

Management and Operation

The multicultural library expects all types of libraries to adopt an integrated service approach. The core activities of library and information services for culturally and linguistically diverse communities are central, not "separate" or "additional," and should always be designed to meet local or specific needs.

The library should have a policy and a strategic plan, defining its mission, objectives, priorities and services related to cultural diversity. The plan should be based on a comprehensive user needs analysis and adequate resources.

Library activities should not be developed in isolation. Cooperation with relevant user groups and professionals at local, national or international level should be encouraged.

Core Actions

The multicultural library should:

- develop culturally diverse and multilingual collections and services, including digital and multimedia resources;
- allocate resources for the preservation of cultural expression and heritage, paying particular attention to oral, indigenous and intangible cultural heritage;
- include programmes supporting user education, information literacy skills, newcomer resources, cultural heritage and cross-cultural dialogue as integral parts of the services;
- provide access to library resources in appropriate languages through information organization and access systems;
- develop marketing and outreach materials in appropriate media and languages to attract different groups to the library.

Staff

The library staff is the active intermediary between users and resources. Professional education and continuing training focused on services to multicultural communities, cross-cultural communication and sensitivity, anti-discrimination, cultures and languages should be provided.

The staff of a multicultural library should reflect the cultural and linguistic characteristic of the community to ensure cultural awareness, reflect the community the library serves, and encourage communication.

Funding, Legislation and Networks

Governments and other relevant decision-making bodies are urged to establish and adequately fund libraries and library systems to offer free library and information services to culturally diverse communities.

Multicultural library services are in essence global. All libraries involved in activities in this field must participate in relevant local, national or international networks in policy development. Research is needed to obtain the data necessary to make informed service decisions and secure appropriate funding. Research findings and best practices should be widely disseminated in order to guide effective multicultural library services.

Implementing the Manifesto

The international community must recognize and support libraries and information services in their role of promoting and preserving cultural and linguistic diversity.

Decision makers at all levels and the library community around the world are hereby requested to disseminate this Manifesto and to carry out the principles and actions expressed herein. (March 2012)

***To access the document online, follow: https://www.ifla.org/files/assets/library-services-to-multicultural-populations/publications/multicultural_library_manifesto-en.pdf

This manifesto makes an extremely important point when it states, "The core activities of library and information services for culturally and linguistically diverse communities are *central*, not '*separate*' or '*additional*,' and should always be designed to meet local or specific needs" (author's italics). And, of course, this concept must be extended to the LGBTQ population.

There is also available an "IFLA/UNESCO Multicultural Library Manifesto Toolkit," which was developed to give practical approaches to libraries on how to apply the concepts in the manifesto and includes an "Implementation Kit," "Community Analysis and Needs Assessment," "Developing a Mission Statement," "Understanding the Manifesto: Workshop Handbook," and "Core Actions—Toolkit Checklist" (https://www.ifla.org/node/8977).

CONSUMER HEALTH INFORMATION FOR NON-ENGLISH SPEAKERS

The good news is that there is an abundance of sources for information for the non-English speaker; the vast majority of it is free and readily available on the internet. NNLM, in collaboration with the NNLM Consumer Outreach Librarians, offers a pathfinder, "Consumer Health Information in Many Languages Resources" (https://nnlm.gov/consumer-health-information-many-languages-resources), which includes the following sources:

- MedlinePlus Health Information in Multiple Languages (http://www.nlm.nih.gov/medlineplus/languages/languages.html). Information in more than forty-six languages. The entire site is also in both English and Spanish.
- Consumer Health Information in Many Languages Resources, a collaboration of the NNLM Consumer Outreach Librarians (https://nnlm.gov/consumer-health-information-many-languages-resources). This wonderful resource directs patrons to multilanguage sources of information in specific areas, including a section on "Resources for Specific Languages."
- Cancer Index (http://www.cancerindex.org/clinks13.htm). Languages include Dutch, Finnish, French, German, Greek, Japanese, and Spanish.
- EthnoMed (http:ethnomed.org). EthnoMed contains information about cultural beliefs, medical issues and related topics pertinent to the health care of immigrants to the US, many of whom are refugees fleeing war-torn parts of the world. Languages include Amharic, Cambodian, Chinese, Eritrean, Ethiopian, and Spanish.
- Health Information Translations (https://www.healthinformationtranslations.org). A collaborative project of four health systems in central Ohio, this site offers culturally appropriate easy-to-read materials, searchable by keyword, health topic, language, and multimedia resources.

- HealthReach (https://healthcare.nlm.nih.gov). HealthReach is a national collaborative partnership that has created a resource of quality multilingual, multicultural public health information for those working with or providing care to individuals with limited English proficiency.
- Hmong Health Website (http://www.hmonghealth.org). The goal of Hmong Health Education Network's website is to provide access to health information for Hmong people and those who provide health, education, and social services to the Hmong community. NLM provides funding.
- SPIRAL: Selected Patient Information Resources in Asian Languages (http://spiral.tufts.edu). Consumer health information in several Asian languages, including Cambodian Khmer, Chinese, Hmong Hmoob, Japanese, Korean, and Vietnamese.
- Health Information in Multiple Languages (https://www.nimhd.nih.gov/programs/edutraining/language-access/health-information/). From the National Institute on Minority Health and Health Disparities. Topics include cancer, diabetes, cardiovascular disease, HIV/AIDS, and immunizations.
- Publications in other Languages from the FDA (https://www.fda.gov/InternationalPrograms/FDAPublicationsinForeignLanguages/). A wide variety of topics in a number of languages.

And don't forget: It would be a wonderful idea, perhaps even a necessity, to hire employees that are fluent in English and the non-English language most prevalent in the library's community.

MULTICULTURAL CONSUMER HEALTH INFORMATION

- The NNLM Middle Atlantic Region "Multicultural Health Information Resources" from the Division of Specialized Information Services (SIS) is a great place to start (https://nnlm.gov/mar/guides/multicultural).
- Minority Health Information Outreach (https://sis.nlm.nih.gov/outreach/minorityhealth_outreach.html). Information on specific minority populations and minority health educational materials.
- Arctic Health (https://arctichealth.nlm.nih.gov). The Arctic Health website is a central source for information on diverse aspects of the Arctic environment and the health of northern peoples. The site gives access to evaluated health information from hundreds of local, state, national, and international agencies, as well as from professional societies and universities.
- American Indian Health (https://americanindianhealth.nlm.nih.gov/). This web resource on American Indian Health, sponsored by the National Library of Medicine, is designed to bring together health and medical resources pertinent to the American Indian population including policies, consumer health infor-

mation, and research. Links are provided here to an assortment of documents, websites, databases, and other resources.
- Native Hawaiian and Pacific Islander Health (https://medlineplus.gov/native hawaiianandpacificislanderhealth.html). Links to health issues that affect Native Hawaiians and Pacific Islanders, including specific diseases (e.g., cancer, chronic liver disease, diabetes, heart disease); women's health; and "Find an Expert." Information in Chamorro, Chuukese, Marshallese, Samoan, Tagalog, and Tongan.
- MedlinePlus pages. Always remember MedlinePlus as a source of information! including the following:
  - Health Disparities (https://medlineplus.gov/healthdisparities.html)
  - African American Health (https://medlineplus.gov/africanamericanhealth.html)
  - Asian American Health (https://medlineplus.gov/asianamericanhealth.html)
  - Hispanic American Health (https://medlineplus.gov/hispanicamericanhealth.html)

And don't forget: Regarding programming, heed the advice of Walker and Polepeddi when they recommend presenting library programs bilingually. "Delivering programs in the home language is another way a library signals its commitment to serving a particular population. Having a program delivered in the nondominant language sometimes creates tension in a library community" (2013, 11).

The influx of immigrants from all parts of the world makes it necessary for libraries to have health information not only in languages other than English, but also information that explains how different customs, religions, cultures, and ethnic groups will impact the health-care experience. As Baughman and Parker pointedly observe: "Assume most of what you know of another culture is not correct, especially if you learned it in a traditional American school or college setting" (2015, 256).

The AHRQ's (2015) "Health Literacy Universal Precautions Toolkit," 2nd ed., offers a list of examples:

- Health beliefs: In some cultures, people believe that talking about a possible poor health outcome will cause that outcome to occur.
- Health customs: In some cultures, family members play a large role in health care decision making.
- Ethnic customs: Differing roles of women and men in society may determine who makes decisions about accepting and following through with medical treatments.
- Religious beliefs: Religious faith and spiritual beliefs may affect health care–seeking behavior and people's willingness to accept specific treatment or behavior changes.

- Dietary customs: Disease-related dietary advice will be difficult to follow if it does not conform to the foods or cooking methods used.
- Interpersonal customs: Eye contact or physical touch will be expected in some cultures and inappropriate or offensive in others.

All librarians and professional library organizations follow a code of ethics that clearly state the profession's commitment to inclusiveness, providing a welcoming environment and free access to all information to all communities. The American Library Association (ALA, n.d.-a) states that "Equity, Diversity and Inclusion are fundamental values of the association and its members, and diversity is listed as one of ALA's Key Action Areas."

Diversity and inclusion are also essential values of the Medical Library Association. With these core values in mind, consumer health information collections need to address the LGBTQ community as a whole and specifically to the needs of individual libraries' communities.

LGBTQ CONSUMER HEALTH INFORMATION

It's a shameful and deplorable fact that some in the LGBTQ community face ignorance, discrimination, hostility, and even violence from others that may even extend to their interactions with clinicians and the health-care system as a whole. This presents barriers to LGBTQ individuals seeking proper and timely health care. In addition, "Studies show conclusively that LGBT teens are routinely bullied, both verbally and physically, harassed, and marginalized by their peers. Such treatment and negative experiences often result in higher rates of depression, suicidal thoughts, suicide attempts, and substance abuse for LGBT teens" (Joseph 2015). Elder LGBTQ persons have their own difficulties including finding clinicians, as well as LGBTQ-friendly nursing and assisted living homes.

Let the library be a place where LGBTQ community members of all ages can find a welcoming, nonjudgmental atmosphere and the health information they need. Both the American Library Association (ALA) and the Medical Library Association (MLA) are on the forefront of striving toward inclusiveness in library collections and service. ALA's website includes a section on "Outreach Resources for Services to Gay, Lesbian, Bisexual, and Transgender People," which offers resources to provide such services. ALA (n.d.-b) points out that while the Library Bill of Rights affirms that all libraries should provide access to information to all people, the GLBT communities' access may be limited by the following factors:

- Collections which don't represent GLBT content or perspectives
- Environments which are not welcoming or inclusive through actions by staff and other patrons
- Services not promoted to GLBT populations or in collaborations with local GLBT organizations

In an EBSCO blog, Stacey (2016) suggests some ideas to increase LGBT patrons' inclusiveness in the library experience:

- Encourage community involvement in collection development
- Participate in Pride celebrations by having book displays or exhibits
- Provide meeting space for LGBT organizations
- Ensure that Pro-LGBT websites are accessible

The following are some resources that will provide libraries with reliable and accurate information:

- MedlinePlus: Gay, Lesbian, Bisexual, and Transgender Health (https://medlineplus.gov/gaylesbianbiseuxalandtransgenderhealth.html)
- CDC: Lesbian, Gay, Bisexual, and Transgender Health (https://www.cdc.gov/lgbthealth/)
- Gay and Lesbian Medical Association (GLMA) (http://www.glma.org). Features include an all-important "Find a Provider," a way to find LGBTQ-friendly clinicians; "10 Things Gay Men Should Discuss with Their Healthcare Providers," "10 Things Lesbians Should Discuss with Their Healthcare Providers," "10 Things Bisexuals Should Discuss with Their Healthcare Providers," and "10 Things Transgender Persons Should Discuss with Their Healthcare Providers."
- American Psychological Association (APA) Lesbian, Gay, Bisexual and Transgender Health (http://www.apa.org/pi/lgbt/resources/lgbt-health.aspx). Information and resources regarding LGBT health disparities and advocacy from the Office on Sexual Orientation and Gender Diversity
- Human Rights Campaign Healthcare Equality Index (http://www.hrc.org/hei/for-lgbt-patients). HRC is the largest civil rights organization working to achieve equality for lesbian, gay, bisexual, transgender, and queer Americans. Their "Healthcare Equality Index" provides resources including sections on "Know Your Healthcare Rights," "Coming Out to Your Doctor," and a link to the GMLA "Find a Provider" page.
- The Fenway Institute National LGBT Health Education Center (https://lgbthealtheducation.org/about-us/lgbt-health-education/). The Fenway Institute works to make life healthier for LGBT people, people living with HIV/AIDS, and the larger community through research and evaluation, education and training, and public health policy. Resources include publications, most of which are freely accessible for download.
- Services & Advocacy for GLBT Elders (SAGE) (http://www.sageusa.org). The country's largest and oldest organization dedicated to improving the lives of LGBT older adults. Resources include publications on health issues.
- Gay-Straight Alliance Network (https://www.gsanetwork.org). A GSA is a student-run club in a high school or middle school that brings together LGBTQ and straight students to support each other, provide a safe place to socialize, and create a platform to fight for racial, gender, LGBTQ, and economic justice. The

GSA Network provides a directory of nationwide GSAs and information and resources on how to establish one.

And don't forget: Be sure to investigate if there are local organizations for referral, for education, and also for possible library partnerships. For example, on Long Island, New York, the LGBT Network (http://lgbtnetwork.org/), is an association of non-profit organizations that work to serve the LGBT community of Long Island and Queens (a borough of NYC) throughout one's life span.

NNLM OUTREACH AND COURSES

Jacqueline Leskovec, network librarian for NNLM Greater Midwest Region (GMR), and Tony Nguyen, technology and communications coordinator, NNLM Southeastern/Atlantic Region (SEA), have written a CE course for librarians, "Improving the Health, Safety and Well-Being of LGBT Populations," and Patricia J. Devine, outreach and communications coordinator for NNLM Pacific Northwest Region (PNR), and Nguyen wrote "LGBT Elder Population Health Awareness." Check the NNLM training schedule (https://nnlm.gov/professional-development) for these and other pertinent courses.

The library serves as an information hub for its community, whether that community is a town, city, university, or hospital or health center. An inviting, welcoming atmosphere is conducive to providing information to all members of the community it serves, and, for that matter, anyone who walks in the door.

REFERENCES

AHRQ (Agency for Healthcare Research and Quality). 2015. "AHRQ Health Literacy Universal Precautions Toolkit." 2nd ed. January 2015. https://www.ahrq.gov/sites/default/files/publications/files/healthlittoolkit2_3.pdf.

ALA (American Library Association). n.d.-a. "Equality, Diversity, and Inclusion." http://www.ala.org/advocacy/diversity.

ALA (American Library Association). n.d.-b. "Outreach Resources for Services to Gay, Lesbian, Bisexual, and Transgender People." http://www.ala.org/advocacy/diversity/outreachtounderservedpopulations/servicesgay.

American Heart Association. 2017. "African-Americans and Heart Disease, Stroke." August 22, 2017. http://www.heart.org/HEARTORG/Conditions/More/MyHeartandStrokeNews/African-Americans-and-Heart-Disease_UCM_444863_Article.jsp#.WVFyi4jyvIU.

Baughman, Kris, and Rebecca Marcum Parker. 2013. "Programs, Signage, and the Kitchen Sink: Attracting Multicultural Patrons to School Libraries." In *Library Service for Multicultural Patrons: Strategies to Encourage Library Use*, edited by Carol Smallwood and Kim Becnel, 243–56. Lanham, MD: Scarecrow Press.

IFLA/UNESCO. 2012. "Multicultural Library Manifesto: The Multicultural Library—A Gateway to a Cultural Diverse Society in Dialogue." March 2012. https://www/ifla.org/files/assets/library-services-to-multicultural-populations/publications/multicultural_library+manifesto-en.pdf.

Indian Health Service. 2017. "Disparities." US Department of Health and Human Services. Indian Health Service: The Federal Health Program for American Indians and Alaska Natives. https://www.ihs.gov/newsroom/factsheets/disparities/.

Joseph, Claire B. 2015. "LGBT Teens and Peer Acceptance." In *Salem Health: Adolescent Health & Wellness*, edited by Paul Moglia, 172–74. Amenia, NY: Grey House.

Pew Research Center. 2016. "Just 10 States Resettled More Than Half of Recent Refugees to the U.S." December 6, 2016. http://www.pewresearch.org/fact-tank/2016/12/06/just-10-states-resettled-more-than-half-of-recent-refugees-to-u-s/.

Stacey, Sandra. 2016. "Is Your Library Doing Enough for LGBT Patrons?" *EBSCO blog*. June 6, 2016. https://www.ebsco.com/blog/article/is-your-library-doing-enough-for-lgbt-patrons.

Walker, Donna, and Padma Polepeddi. 2013. "Becoming a Multicultural Services Library: A Guided Journey to Serving Diverse Populations." In *Library Service for Multicultural Patrons: Strategies to Encourage Library Use*, edited by Carol Smallwood and Kim Becnel, 3–12. Lanham, MD: Scarecrow Press.

10

Where Consumers Go to Find Health Information

Apps, Social Media, and Wikipedia

Takeaways from this chapter:

- *Where people look for health information*
- *How the library can connect with their patrons via social media*
- *How to help patrons make informed choices*
- *What to do if patrons don't accept the librarian's recommendations*

The internet has changed forever how, where, and when people search for information. Any library planning a consumer health information service needs to recognize and fully understand its patrons' use not only of internet search engines and websites, but also of apps, social media, and Wikipedia to find health information. Librarians are in a position to guide their patrons to the best consumer health information, but they must also be prepared for some "pushback" or resistance to their recommendations.

APPS

According to the Pew Research Center (2017), 77 percent of Americans own a smartphone, and while "smartphones are nearly ubiquitous among younger adults, with 92% of 18- to 29-year-olds owning one," "74% of Americans ages 50–64" also own smartphones. In addition, "nearly seven-in-ten Americans now use social media."

A 2015 study by the IMS Institute for Healthcare Informatics found more than 165,000 health-care apps on the Apple iOS and Google app platforms. Over two-thirds are devoted to wellness, including fitness, lifestyle, and diet and nutrition

(IMS Institute for Healthcare Informatics 2015). As Krebs and Duncan (2015) point out, "The field of mobile health apps is still in a nascent stage . . . most health apps have not been designed with input from health care . . . professionals."

The proliferation of health apps, and especially the inflated health improvement claims of some, piqued the Federal Drug Administration (FDA)'s interest. In 2015, the FDA issued a report, in which they separate mobile health apps into two categories. They stated that the "FDA intends to apply its regulatory oversight to only those mobile apps that are medical devices and whose functionality could pose a risk to a patient's safety if the mobile app were to not function as intended" (FDA 2015, 4). Examples include "mobile apps that control medical devices" (FDA 2015, 14) such as blood pressure cuffs and insulin delivery.

The second category is "mobile apps for which FDA intends to exercise enforcement discretion (meaning that FDA does not intend to enforce requirements under the FD&C [Federal, Food, Drug, and Cosmetic] Act)" (FDA 2015, 15) "because they pose a low risk to patients" (16), which includes those that "help patients . . . self-manage their disease or conditions without providing specific treatment or treatment suggestions" (15) and "provide easy access to information related to patients' health conditions or treatments" (15). The report includes extensive lists for apps that fall into both categories.

Librarians may very well be asked by their patrons how to determine if an app is credible. In general, consumers can only rely on "ratings" of other users. In 2015, Stoyanov et al. devised a "Mobile App Rating Scale [MARS]: A New Tool for Assessing the Quality of Health Mobile Apps." In this they discuss their development of this scale (MARS) that "provide[s] a multidimensional measure of the app quality indicators of engagement, functionality, aesthetics, and information quality, as well as app subjective quality."

HealthIT.gov (https://www.healthit.gov) is a national resource on health information technology for consumers and health-care professionals. On their "Patients & Families" section, they offer guidelines on how to "Find Quality Resources" under the "e-Health" tab. (See Sample Form 10.1)

SAMPLE FORM 10.1

HealthIT.gov Guidelines: Find Quality Resources in e-Health

How do I know if I can trust the information I find online? How do I know if an eHealth tool is right for me or for my family?

With thousands of web pages, online services, and apps related to health, it can be hard to find high quality, trusted, relevant resources to meet your needs and the needs of your family.

In some cases you can get trustworthy recommendations from doctors and nurses, from other experts, or from consumer organizations. But when doing your own research, it's in your best interest to look at resources carefully, particularly before making a purchase or making a decision about a health condition.

Here are some questions to consider while you decide whether or not a given tool or resource is right for you.

Is It Up-to-Date?

Generally, web pages will indicate when they were last updated, and apps will indicate when the latest version was released. But even without exact information, you can often make educated guesses about whether or not a resource is up-to-date by looking at the material. For example, if an article about a health condition mentions research from the last five years, it's probably more up-to-date than an article that only mentions research from twenty years ago. But keep in mind that not everything needs to be updated frequently. For example, the science of basic care of cuts and bruises doesn't change much from year to year, or even decade to decade.

Whose Name Is on It and Who Provides It?

Some resources are sponsored or sold by private companies. Others are sold or provided free-of-charge by government offices, non-profit organizations, or educational institutions. One type of sponsorship is not necessarily better than another. But keep in mind that the sponsor of a resource may have an interest or agenda different from your own.

Is the Information Accurate?

While medicine is based on science, some health information on the web and provided through apps may be biased. Consider sources carefully, particularly when they guide you towards specific treatment options or towards a specific product.

For Apps and Devices, Do They Work as Advertised?

More than ever before, people have access to a mix of product reviews written by professionals and by individuals like themselves. Try to find unbiased sources of reviews and read them carefully to learn more about whether or not a product performs as promised, and whether or not it will address the specific needs you have. Also, look for endorsements by professional organizations like medical associations, or certifications by government agencies like the <u>Food and Drug Administration</u>.

Are the Tools or Resources Easily Usable?

On a web site, is it easy to search for the information you need? In an app, is it easy for you to understand how it works and how to use it? If you have a disability, does the resource include accessibility features or work with assistive software?

Does it Work with Other Tools and Resources?

For example, does a device give you choices about what to do with the data it collects, or are you limited to seeing it on the device itself, or just the product's web site? Does a web site that tracks information for you offer ways to connect that information to other resources either automatically or through options to export your information?

Is it Secure? Does it Protect your Privacy?

Any resource that collects personal health information about you or your family can expose you to potential risks. When evaluating such tools, look for privacy and security policies that protect your data and ensure that no one can access your information without your explicit permission. (The Office of the National Coordinator for Health IT (ONC) offers a <u>model privacy policy</u> for companies offering personal health records.)

It should be no surprise that these guidelines are very similar to the Medical Library Association's guidelines on consumer health websites. HealthIT.gov also has a short list, "Access Wellness Resources" (https://www.healthit.gov/patients-families/stay-well), that allows users to learn more about personal wellness devices, wellness apps, and other resources for general wellness information; just a fraction of resources available is listed. The page includes a disclaimer: "The Department of Health and Human Services or the U.S. Government does not endorse any product, service, or general policies of any non-Federal entity nor is responsible for the content of any individual organization's material or web pages found at these links."

An app site that can be recommended to patrons is iMedicalApps.com. Started and maintained by two physicians who lead a team that provide reviews and research, this is the leading online site for medical professionals, patients, and analysts interested in mobile medical technology and health-care apps. The home page includes "Best apps of the month," and it may be searched by specialty and platform. The team is now working on iPrescribeApps.com, a platform that will enable providers to prescribe health apps to their patients.

SOCIAL MEDIA

"Social media" is an umbrella term that includes apps, Facebook, Twitter, YouTube, and Wikipedia. Dalmer observes that "social media's capacity to change the way in which online health information is produced, accessed, trusted, and filtered warrants a greater and more focused examination by information professionals" (2017, 65), announcing a new challenge to create a tool that generates a user-friendly "snapshot" of model privacy practices for digital health products.

Many social media sites serve as avenues for consumers to connect with others who share their health issues in support groups, and to find out individuals' unique and nuanced experiences. This is a vital element of the health-care continuum that cannot be downplayed. However, it remains incumbent on consumer health librarians to urge caution with the reliability of information offered.

A 2012 study from PricewaterhouseCoopers' Health Research Institute states that "age is the most influential factor in engaging and sharing through social media. More than 80% of individual ages 18–24 would be likely to share health information . . . 45% of individuals ages 45–64 would be likely to share via social media." Astonishingly, "90% of individuals would . . . trust information found via social media" (PwC Health Research Institute 2012). Librarians are in a powerful position to educate patrons on the discriminating use of social media for health issues.

How Libraries Can Use Social Media

Every library should be part of the social media scene. Public libraries need to be on Facebook and Twitter; many, if not most, are. Posts should be done daily. This is a great way to get the message across to a large population. As the CDC (2012) points out, social media helps organizations achieve their goals; to paraphrase them:

- Engage with the library's patrons.
- Personalize health messages and target them to a particular audience.
- Alert patrons to upcoming programming.
- Empower people to make safer and healthier decisions.

Each library should develop a social media policy and guidelines for their employees and designate an employee to be the administrator of the social media accounts. One good example of policy and guidelines is from the Health Sciences Library Association of New Jersey (HSLANJ, n.d.). Part of this is shown below.

> The Health Sciences Library Association of New Jersey (HSLANJ) recognizes the importance of online social tools for communication with members, prospective members, sponsors, members of the medical and allied health communities and the general public and the general public. The guidelines below will help open up a respectful interaction with people on the Internet while protecting the privacy, confidentiality, and mission of HSLANJ and its members. HSLANJ's social media sites are designed to serve as a forum for interaction. HSLANJ encourages discussions, comments and questions related to both the profession and the organization. All official Forums must be monitored periodically by an administrator who has the authority to remove content that violates these guidelines.
>
> 1. Identify yourself—State your name and, when relevant, role at HSLANJ—when discussing HSLANJ or HSLANJ-related matters.
> 2. Be responsible for what you write.
> 3. Be authentic.
> 4. Consider your audience.
> 5. Exercise good judgment.
> 6. Respect copyrights and fair use.
> 7. Remember to protect confidential & proprietary info.
> 8. Bring value to the posts that you make.

A 2016 report from the Pew Research Center, *Hispanic Trends*, states that "overall, 80% of Latino adults . . . access the internet via a mobile device such as a cell phone or tablet . . . nearly all 18- to 29-year-old Latinos (94%) and 30- to 49-year-old Latinos (89%) use the internet on a mobile device" (Pew Research Center 2016a). With this high smartphone use, a library might consider alerting Latino consumers about health programming via emails or Twitter. Of course, the library would first have to obtain emails or Twitter accounts, but this could be accomplished in a number of ways, including reaching out to the community at a hospital or community organization health fair, and creating a public event, maybe a library QR code—perhaps one that displays an interactive library Facebook "like" button—that fair participants could scan onto their mobile devices.

Barbakoff and Gomez suggest building a Latino-centric mobile app; libraries can consider two major design features (based on advertising studies): interactive or media and culturally relevant content that clearly targets Latinos (2013, 198).

WIKIPEDIA

In 2015, in the English-language version of Wikipedia, there were 97.2 billion page views, and "Wikipedia is the leading single source of healthcare information for patients and healthcare professionals." Yes, astonishingly, health-care professionals, too! It is also important to note that "in Google, at least one Wikipedia page will be displayed among the first ten results in a staggering 84% of all medically-related search queries" (Pew Research Center 2016b). Wikipedia is a force to be reckoned with, and it has its staunch supporters. So what's the problem with turning to Wikipedia for health information? Librarians need to be able to answer that question!

Wikipedia has actively reached out to several professional communities. In fact, in 2012, Wikimedia founded "WikiProject Med (WPMEDF)" (https://meta.wikimedia.org/wiki/Wiki_Project_Med), which in part sought to form collaborations with medical schools, to "provide the sum of all medical knowledge to all people in their own language" (Wikimedia and Wikipedia are interrelated). Azzam et al., in their study "Why Medical Schools Should Embrace Wikipedia," reported that the University of California, San Francisco, "had created . . . the first formal medical school course worldwide through which medical students actively work to improve Wikipedia's health-related articles" for academic credit (2017). In addition, "the New York State Health Foundation funded a two-year collaboration between Consumers Union and New York State medical schools to launch the Wikipedia Medical School Project, a pilot that uses medical students as fact checkers and editors to improve the quality and accuracy of Wikipedia's health information" (Byrd 2014).

With regard to Wikipedia's reliability in health information, different studies come to different conclusions. The author had a recent experience where a hospital resident physician insisted that Wikipedia's drug information is just as accurate and reliable as that of Lexicomp, a fee-based online database that provides point-of-care drug information for clinicians, including dosage, administration, and warnings (http://www.wolterskluwercdi.com/lexicomp-online/); when the author related this to a hospital pharmacist, the pharmacist was speechless. The study cited by the resident concluded that "Wikipedia is an accurate and comprehensive source of drug-related information for undergraduate medical education" (Kraenbring et al. 2014). Now this may be saying that for a student, the information is fine, but, what about for practicing clinicians?

A study published in the *Journal of the American Pharmacists Association* (Reilly et al. 2017) stated emphatically that "Wikipedia lacks the accuracy and completeness of standard clinical references and should not be a routine part of clinical decision making"; another study (Koppen, Phillips, and Papageorgiou 2015) concluded that "Wikipedia . . . may not be a reliable, up-to-date resource for drug safety information."

Wikipedia is an extremely well-known and popular site for information seekers. But do librarians want to refer their patrons to sites where the information *might* be accurate? Fortunately there is such an abundance of accurate, reliable, up-to-date consumer health information, for all members of any library's community, that there really is no need to refer to Wikipedia. Librarians should recommend the many readily available resources there are.

GENERAL MEDIA

Of course, many consumers learn about health issues from traditional media outlets, including newspapers, both in print and online, and television, including advertisements. When a celebrity suffers a specific ailment, or undergoes surgery, there is immense media coverage and subsequent social media buzz resulting in many seeking information on the topic.

In 2013 actress Angelina Jolie tested positive for the BRCA gene and subsequently decided to undergo a preventive mastectomy; she then wrote a *New York Times* editorial endorsing BRCA testing. As a result, there was an immediate increase in BRCA testing rates (Desai et al. 2016).

The United States and New Zealand share the dubious distinction of being the only countries in the world that allow direct-to-consumer advertising of prescription drugs (AMA 2015). As a result, many consumers will look for information on these drugs and the health issues they are meant to treat. In addition, advertisements can result in increased drug sales, for as Appleby (2017) observes, "Commercials have raised awareness of diseases patients may not know they have."

Librarians need to be proactive and make sure they are aware of "hot" health topics that consumers may very well seek information about. Subscribe to the MedlinePlus Twitter feed that provides links to a wide variety of health-related articles and also to the National Institutes of Health (NIH) "News in Health" monthly newsletter that provides practical health news and tips based on NIH research (https://www.nih.gov/health-information).

STAY THE COURSE AND KEEP THE FAITH

Consumer health librarians have a veritable treasure chest of reliable and easily accessible health information for all their customers, so it can be disappointing and even frustrating to know that patrons are instead turning to information sources that can be incorrect or even suspect. To add to this frustration, a 2016 study showed that consumers value a site's perceived ease of use over its trustworthiness; presumably, consumers' familiarity with a site and comfort level also come into play (Rosin 2016).

Even more disconcerting is an experience Kelli Ham, consumer health librarian for NNLM Pacific Southwest Region, related to the author. In her outreach programs, Kelli will, of course, recommend government-based websites. A few times, people have expressed their distrust of anything related to the government, but on one occasion a gentleman went so far as to say that not only did he not trust anything from the government, but that he trusted WebMD because, as a for-profit company, they cared if he lived or died. Librarians need to model themselves after Kelli Ham and remain professional and nonjudgmental as she did in this situation regardless of her differing opinion on the matter (Kelli Ham, personal communication with author, May 30, 2017).

Consumer health librarians have the opportunity to educate and enlighten their customers and help them to learn more about their health issues and ultimately empower themselves in their navigation through the health-care system. This does not mean that every patron encounter will be met with enthusiasm or agreement, but this should not and cannot discourage librarians in their overall mission.

REFERENCES

AMA (American Medical Association). 2015. "AMA Calls for Ban on DTC Ads of Prescription Drugs and Medical Devices." Press release, November 17, 2015. https://www.ama-assn.org/content/ama-calls-ban-direct-consumer-advertising-prescription-drugs-and-medical-devices#.

Appleby, Julie. 2017. "Ad for Anti-crying Drug Sends Sales Soaring." *New York Times*, May 14, 2017. https://www.nytimes.com/2017/05/12/business/media/pseudobulbar-affect-drug-advertising-sales.html.

Azzam, Amin, David Bresler, Armando Leon, Lauren Maggio, et al. 2017. "Why Medical Schools Should Embrace Wikipedia: Final-Year Medical Student Contributions to Wikipedia Articles for Academic Credit at One School." *Academic Medicine* 92, no. 2: 194–200. doi.10.1097/ACM.0000000000001381.

Barbakoff, Audrey, and Kristina Gomez. 2013. "Virtual Services to Latinos and Spanish Speakers." In *Library Services for Multicultural Patrons: Strategies to Encourage Library Use*, edited by Carol Smallwood and Kim Becnel, 193–202. Lanham, MD: Scarecrow Press.

Byrd, Brian. 2014. "Improving the Accuracy of Wikipedia's Medical Information." *Health Affairs Blog*. December 9, 2014. http://healthaffairs.org/blog/2014/12/09/improving-the-accuracy-of-wikipedias-medical-information.

CDC (Centers for Disease Control and Prevention). 2012. *CDC's Guide to Writing for Social Media*. US Department of Health and Human Services. https://www.cdc.gov/socialmedia/tools/guidelines/pdf/guidetowritingforsocialmedia.pdf.

Dalmer, Nicole K. 2017. "Questioning Reliability Assessments of Health Information on Social Media." *Journal of the Medical Library Association* 105, no. 1 (January): 61–68. doi:10.5195/jmla2017.108.

Desai, Sunita, Marshall J. Seidman, Anupam B. Jena, and Ruth L. Newhouse. 2016. "Do Celebrity Endorsements Matter? Observational Study of BRCA Gene Testing and Mastectomy Rates after Angelina Jolie's *New York Times* Editorial." *British Medical Journal* 355, no. i6357. doi:10.1136/bmj.i6357.

FDA (Food and Drug Administration). 2015. *Mobile Medical Applications: Guidance for Industry and Food and Drug Administration Staff.* February 9, 2015. US Department of Health and Human Services, Food and Drug Administration Center for Devices and Radiological Health/Center for Biologics Evaluation and Research. https:www/fda/gov/downloads/MedicalDevices/DeviceRegulationandGuidance/GuidanceDocuments/UCM263366.pdf. Accessed June 23, 2017.

HSLANJ (Health Sciences Library Association of New Jersey). n.d. "Social Media Guidelines." http://hslanj.org/resources/social-media-guidelines/.

IMS Institute for Healthcare Informatics. 2015. "Patient Adoption of mHealth: Use, Evidence and Remaining Barriers to Mainstream Acceptance." September 2015. http://www.imshealth.com/files/web/IMSH%20Institute/Reports/Patient%20Adoption%20of%20mHealth/IIHI_Patient_Adoption_of_mHealth.pdf.

Koppen, Laura, Jennifer Phillips, and Renee Papageorgiou. 2015. "Analysis of Reference Sources Used in Drug-Related Wikipedia Articles." *Journal of the Medical Library Association* 103, no. 3 (July): 140–44.

Kraenbring, Jona, Tika Monzon Penza, Joanna Gutmann, Susanne Muehlich, et al. 2014. "Accuracy and Completeness of Drug Information in Wikipedia: A Comparison with Standard Textbooks of Pharmacology." *PLOS One* 9, no. 9 (September): e106930. doi:10.1371/journal.pone.0106930.

Krebs, Paul, and Dustin T. Duncan. 2015. "Health App Use among US Mobile Phone Owners: A National Survey." *JMIR mHealth uHealth* 3, no. 4: e101. doi:10.2196/mhealth.4924.

Pew Research Center. 2016a. *Hispanic Trends: Hispanics and Mobile Access to the Internet.* July 20, 2016. http://www.pewhispanic.org/2016/07/20/3-hispanics-and-mobile-access-to-the-internet/.

Pew Research Center. 2016b. "Wikipedia at 15: Millions of Readers in Scores of Languages." January 24, 2016. http://www.pewresearch.org/fact-tank/2016/01/14/Wikipedia-at-15/.

Pew Research Center. 2017. "Record Shares of Americans Now Own Smartphones, Have Home Broadband." January 12, 2017. www.pewresearch.org/fact-tank/2017/01/12/evolution-of-technology/.

PwC Health Research Institute. 2012. "Social Media 'Likes' Healthcare: From Marketing to Social Business." https://www.pwc.com/us/en/health-industries/health-research-institute/publications/pdf/health-care-social-media-report.pdf.

Reilly, Timothy, William Jackson, Victoria Berger, and Danielle Candelario. 2017. "Accuracy and Completeness of Drug Information in Wikipedia Medication Monographs." *Journal of the American Pharmacists Association* 57, no. 2: 193–96. http://dx.doi.org/10.1016/j.japh.2016.10.007.

Rosin, Tamara. 2016. "Consumers Value Ease of Use over Trust When Seeking Healthcare Information." *Becker's Hospital Review*, March 10, 2016. http://www.beckershospitalreview

.com/hospital-management-administration/consumers-value-ease-of-use-over-trust-when-seeking-healthcare-information.html.

Stoyanov, Stoyan R., Leanne Hides, David J. Kavanagh, Oksana Zelenko, et al. 2015. "Mobile App Rating Scale: A New Tool for Assessing the Quality of Health Mobile Apps." *JMIR mHealth uHealth* 3, no. 1: e27. doi:10.2196/mhealth.3422.

WikiProjectMed (WPMEDF). https://meta.wikimedia.org/wiki/Wiki_Project_Med.

11

Consumer Health Information Outreach for Every Library

Takeaways from this chapter:

- *How any library of any size and any budget can provide outreach*
- *How to take the library into the community*

The number of consumer health library outreach programs, or community partnerships with the aim of linking library patrons with excellent health information tailored to their needs, is amazing. Never underestimate the ingenuity, creativity, initiative, and dedication of librarians to help their customers in the best way possible.

As previously noted, it would take multiple volumes to list all of the outstanding programs initiated; the following will highlight a sampling of programming not previously mentioned. An important concept to remember is that any activity or initiative that gets authoritative and reliable consumer health information into a customer's hands is to be celebrated. As community outreach programs begin with community needs assessments and often partnerships with community groups that have been identified as in need of specific health information, this will explore a wide variety of outreach programs, including low tech and low cost.

COMMUNITY OUTREACH

There's nothing more low tech and low (or no) cost with respect to a consumer outreach initiative than having a presence at a community event. Even if the event is not specifically related to health, such as a street fair, the library can still make its presence known. All this needs is a table, a librarian, and some free literature to distribute. However, even with such a humble outreach, the rewards can be great.

The hospital where the author works, South Nassau Communities Hospital, a 455-bed teaching, community hospital in suburban Oceanside, Long Island, New York, has an annual 5K race for fund-raising (usually earmarked for some hospital center; in 2016 the proceeds went to the hospital's Feil Cancer Center). Along with the race, the hospital holds a health fair for participants and the community at large. A wide variety of hospital departments is represented with a wide variety of information. In addition, resident physicians and nurses check blood pressure and offer other health screenings.

The author participates by setting up a table with consumer health information. Handouts are all collected free of charge via the library's NNLM, namely, the Middle Atlantic Region (MAR). MAR provides, on their website, sources to contact for (mostly) free materials (https://nnlm.gov/mar/guides/consumer-health/materials), some of which are listed below. In addition, there is a link to an online form to order free NLM materials (https://nnlm.gov/mar/order), some of which are suitable for consumers. A MedlinePlus bookmark in English and Spanish is an effective giveaway; its size is conducive to acceptance, as some people at the health fair don't want to walk away loaded with materials.

And don't expect people to stop by your table automatically. Make a point to say hello to everyone that passes, and call them over to your table. The consumer health items on the table are meant to be *given away*, not repacked and returned to the library! Sometimes some additional giveaways, such as candy, will get people to the table. Another option is to purchase some sort of "prize" to give away; it need not be big or expensive. In the past the author has purchased a small gift bag of toiletries for no more than $15 and raffled it off. Almost everyone will stop to fill out a raffle ticket for a prize, or take free candy; in this way they've stopped at the table and the librarian can hand them consumer health material and tell them about it while they're filling out their raffle or munching their goodies (or both). Another added plus is that the raffle tickets can be counted to see how many people stopped by.

Some Free Materials

MedlinePlus Magazine

Libraries can order this in bulk (https://medlineplus.gov/magazine/subscribe.html).

Mental Health

The National Institute of Mental Health (NIMH), part of the National Institutes of Health, offers a variety of free pamphlets in both English and Spanish. Topics include autism, bipolar disease, depression, and suicide prevention, and publications specifically about children and teens (https://www.nimh.nih.gov/health/publications/index.shtml).

Nutrition

The National Heart, Lung, and Blood Institute (NHLBI), part of the National Institutes of Health's "We Can!" program, which provides ways to enhance children's activity and nutrition, offers a variety of free materials for parents, teens, and children available in English and Spanish, some geared for ethnically diverse populations (https://www.nhlbi.nih.gov/health/educational/wecan/).

Diabetes, Digestive Diseases, Kidney Disease, Weight Control, Nutrition, and Obesity

The National Institute of Diabetes and Digestive and Kidney Diseases (NIDDK) of the National Institutes of Health has a wide variety of free materials in both English and Spanish, including a section specifically for "Community Outreach & Health Fairs" (https://www.niddk.nih.gov/health-information/community-outreach-health-fairs).

For Seniors

Go for Life (https://go4life.nia.nih.gov/). An exercise and physical activity campaign from the National Institute on Aging at the National Institutes of Health.

For Kids and Teens

KidsHealth in the Classroom (https://classroom.kidshealth.org/). An offshoot of the excellent KidsHealth website from Nemours. Lots of interesting materials, in both English and Spanish, for kids grades K–12.

Substance Abuse

National Institute on Alcohol Abuse and Alcoholism (NIAAA) of the National Institutes of Health (https://pubs.niaaa.nih.gov/). Wide variety of free publications in English and Spanish. Also see National Institute on Drug Abuse (NIDA) of the National Institutes of Health (https://www.drugabuse.gov/). Variety of publications for all ages; some in Spanish.

Hearing

It's a Noisy Planet from the National Institute on Deafness and Other Communication Disorders of the National Institutes of Health (https://www.noisyplanet.nidcd.nih.gov/). Free publications for all ages in English and Spanish.

Dental Health

National Institute of Dental and Craniofacial Research of the National Institutes of Health (NIDCR) (https://www.nidcr.nih.gov/). Free publications on a variety of topics for all ages, in English and Spanish and some for specific ethnic groups.

As part of their commitment to community health outreach, hospitals are eager potential partners for public libraries. Many hospitals will send different health professionals to public libraries to speak on different health issues; for example, a nurse can speak to a seniors group on Alzheimer's, arthritis, how to prevent falls, and so forth.

Hospitals also routinely make their presence known in the aforementioned community street fairs offering, say, blood pressure screening and literature. In addition, community groups often contact hospitals to speak at their meetings on subjects of importance to them. The hospital where the author works was approached by a church in one of the communities it serves; the church membership was almost exclusively African American, and they wanted the hospital to offer lectures and literature on diseases that disproportionately affect African Americans, for example, heart disease and sickle-cell anemia.

For a few years hospital, South Nassau Communities Hospital had a Sunday morning half-hour radio program, *One Healthy Way* ("One Healthy Way" is the address the hospital created after a large expansion project), that broadcast on a local Long Island, New York, radio station. The author was invited to be the guest five times between 2001 and 2003; each time the topic covered was online consumer health, each show focusing on one specific subject area, for example, men's health, women's health, and so forth.

The University of Virginia (UVA) celebrated the second anniversary of its consumer health information service in early 2017. The "Patient and Family Library" (PFL) space in the *hospital lobby* (author's italics) (the perfect place!) was opened in March 2015 complete with a full-time consumer health librarian, Lydia Witman (Witman 2016). UVA's Claude Moore Health Sciences Library partnered with Medical Center leadership to launch the space and service. Outreach efforts and partnerships in the community include teaching Department of Health community health workers about health literacy and how to find good health information. There are monthly story times for children with "Briar the Book Fair" and monthly health displays coordinated with national observances.

Rochester General Hospital in Rochester, New York, started the "Health Information Ambassador Program." This was modeled after Jackie Davis's (2013) initiative at Sharp HealthCare in San Diego, California. The Werner Medical Library at Rochester General Hospital partnered with the hospital's Volunteer Office to pilot the HIA program on a cardiology inpatient unit. Hospital administrators identified the unit as a priority because of the high volume of patient surveys returned per year and because the unit provides care for a high number of patients with congestive heart failure (CHF) and CHF has one of the highest readmission rates. Readmission rates of recently discharged patients is the bane of any hospital; and getting patients to complete surveys is always a challenge. Elizabeth Mamo, library director of the Werner Medical Library, and Mary Ann Howie, senior librarian, modeled the pilot after a similar program at Cushman Health Library at Sharp Memorial Hospital in San Diego, California (Mamo and Howie 2017). The Volunteer Office assigned volunteers as patient/family experience ambassadors. The consumer health librarian trained volunteers to conduct a reference interview and to address issues pertaining to health literacy. The volunteers round three days per week to offer patients information on their condition or treatment and collect requests. The librarian selects reliable and appropriate material and delivers the information to the patient. As of June 30, 2016, fifteen of the eighty-eight patients completed and returned a hospital survey. Four months of patient satisfaction data show that patients who received assistance through the HIA program reported a significantly better patient experience than those patients who did not receive health information assistance through this program. Specifically, patients who received our service gave a rating in the 99th percentile for both overall rating of the hospital and the willingness to recommend Rochester General Hospital. Patients who did not receive our service rated their experience at around the 50th percentile in the nation. Such survey results are "music to the ears" of administration! Not only does a program like this help patients and their families, but it also offers proof positive of the medical library's value to the hospital's administration.

Akron Children's Hospital's Louis Lame Family Resource Center in Akron, Ohio, provides pediatric consumer health library services for patients, families, health professionals, service provider agencies, and the community. It's located off the Atrium Lobby (great place if you can get it!). One of their outreach initiatives is creating health education lesson plan (H.E.L.P.) kits for school, hospital, and community use (Griggs 2017). Some kits were in collaboration with the local PBS station; others were developed with the assistance of the hospital's subject specialists. Topics include: asthma, dental care, diabetes, hand washing, nutrition, safety, smoking, and teaching tolerance. Each kit is assigned an age group, and the kit will include DVDs, books, puppets, and games in a sturdy plastic file box with a handle. Kits circulate for two weeks. Presentation sites have included Boy and Girl Scout troop meetings, child care centers, and juvenile detention centers.

Tuality Healthcare Library in Hillsboro, Oregon, is a free resource to help the community find answers to their medical and health questions, with personalized support from health information professionals. It's located on the first floor of the Tuality Community Hospital, near the café (another great location!). In partnership with the Washington County Cooperative Library Services (www.wccls.org), patients and the public can check out materials. The library items will be delivered to the hospital for pickup. In addition, medical librarian Judith Hayes has taught a class, "Finding Health Information Online," to librarians throughout Washington County for more than fifteen years (Tuality Healthcare 2016, 3).

Trinitas Regional Medical Center, in Elizabeth, New Jersey, created an online health literacy site that offers quizzes, in English and Spanish, on the topics of stroke, heart attack, medical terminology, Alzheimer's, and prediabetes (http://www.trinitashospital.org/library_health_literacy.htm). Since its inception more than 8,500 people have played, and according to a posttest quiz, 80 percent of participants stated that they will use the information they learned for their health-care decisions (Marrapodi 2016).

PARTNERSHIPS

Berkeley College School of Health Studies in Newark, New Jersey, collaborated with the Newark Public Library to host health fairs in honor of National High Blood Pressure Education Month in May 2017; the program was organized by Laurie McFadden, director of the Berkeley College Newark Campus Library (McFadden 2017). Faculty and students of Berkeley offered free blood pressure screenings, and the library staff provided articles from the MedlinePlus databases in both English and Spanish. And a representative from Whole Foods Market distributed free, healthy snacks. It was one of the library's most popular programs ever.

East Carolina University's Laupus Library is an academic health sciences library that serves the Division of Health Sciences in Greenville, North Carolina. The Laupus Library set strategic goals to serve the citizens of eastern North Carolina to meet their consumer health information needs. In partnership with Sheppard Memorial, the main library for the countywide library system and the city of Greenville, the outreach librarian contacted public library directors in other counties to offer to partner with them to teach consumer health classes to the public in one-hour sessions.

Another partner was Terri Ottosen, consumer health outreach coordinator at NNLM's Southeastern/Atlantic Region (SEA) who gave permission to use an existing course "Prescription for Success: Consumer Health Information" as a template; the Laupus course was named "Healthier U @ Your Library/Hospital." In a "train the trainer" approach, Healthier U sessions were offered in the region's hospitals, which then allowed hospital outreach departments to offer consumer health information training to their communities. The program proved to be a worthwhile effort, ultimately allowing librarians to understand better what their communities need in health information, and in providing rural, underserved populations with training (Coghill and Andresen 2015).

The Suffolk Cooperative Library System, Suffolk County, Long Island, New York, formed a new committee in 2016, the Health Awareness Through Library Outreach (HATLO) Committee. Members include representatives from various county agencies, nonprofit organizations, and libraries to discuss and implement effective methods of sharing up-to-date health-care information through public libraries. In addition, the committee will also focus on all aspects of health literacy and how to create a health-literate society.

SPECIAL POPULATIONS

The Texas Medical Center (TMC) Library provides consumer health information to inmates in forty-five prisons across Texas via the US mail. From 1991 to 2016 the TMC was the regional medical library for the NNLM South Central Region and was assigned to serve as the primary resource for letters regarding consumer health information requests from inmates in state prisons. On average the library received three to five letters per month. "Policies and procedures for answering these letters was minimal but included" information from basic consumer health resources such as MedlinePlus and a standard consumer health disclaimer (Couvillon and Justice 2016, 281). In addition, the librarians responding to the letter were not to sign their name so as to depersonalize the service. "Inmates often share a significant amount of personal information in the form of emotional details about their prison experience and even about the crimes they committed" (281–82). The librarians did not want to convey the idea or encourage a sense that they would or could potentially become the inmate's "pen pal."

A content analysis was performed and included such information as what topic or type of information was requested, and from which unit. The majority of requests were for overviews of a disease or drug. Such requests offered "insight into the health information of a unique population" (285). As Couvillon and Justice conclude, "By providing accurate understandable health information, librarians can offer a valuable service and empower inmates to make better health decisions" (286).

Libraries around the country, alone or in partnerships, proactively work to improve the health of all their patrons by education and services that ultimately allow them to become empowered in just this way. Another great example is the "Library Nurse" program at the Pima County Public Library in Tucson, Arizona. Through a partnership with the Pima County Health Department, a team of public health nurses make rounds in their branch libraries providing basic health services including nursing assessment, nutrition and health education, resource information, and blood pressure screenings; one public health nurse works full-time in the library (Pima County Public Library 2017). In this way the homeless are able to access health services and health information.

THINKING OUTSIDE THE (LUNCH) BOX

It's a shocking and disgraceful fact that in the United States today, more than thirteen million children face hunger, as they live in "food-insecure" households. Good nutrition is particularly important for children whose bodies and organs are developing, especially in the first three years of life. Lack of proper nutrition can be devastating for children in the long term, as it can negatively affect their future physical and mental health (Feeding America 2017).

Some children are fortunate enough to be able to obtain at least one (or maybe two) nutritious meals per day when they are in school. But what happens when schools are in recess for the summer? Public libraries around the country have (quite literally) stepped up to the plate and organized with their local city, county, or state governments to be one of a number of community locations where children can receive breakfast and lunch during summer months. These programs require coordination with the local school system, the USDA, and possibly organizations that may want to cosponsor the event.

One such program is operated in Queens, New York; in partnership with the New York City Board of Education, they offered free lunch for all children under the age of eighteen from June 29 through September 1, 2017, at a number of their branch libraries (Queens Library, n.d.). Another such program is the Henry County Library System in Georgia; they offered free summer lunches to all children under eighteen from June 5 through July 31, 2017, at five branch libraries (Henry County Library System 2017). After enjoying a nutritious and delicious meal, children could take part in fun and free activities at the library, including reading programs and consumer health informational initiatives.

Programs such as these allow the library to serve their communities in very tangible ways. They are quite literally feeding children's bodies and minds. In addition, they are creating tremendous goodwill in their communities, and maybe even introducing the library to children and their families who might otherwise never go there (or even know about it).

Librarians face many challenges in their quest to provide accurate and reliable health information for the communities they serve. Society's pervasive mind-set that the internet and "Dr. Google" are easily navigable without any intermediary assistance—namely, librarians—is especially troubling as there is a real problem with health literacy and with the difficulties faced in attempting to navigate today's increasingly complex health-care system. In addition, there is a significant segment of the population that are medically underserved, with little or no access to adequate health care, let alone adequate health information.

Librarians must be standard bearers in providing accurate and reliable health information for their communities. They are certainly up to the task! There is no end to the amazing ingenuity, creativity, innovation, and resourcefulness of librarians in their initiatives to connect consumer health information with their patrons.

REFERENCES

Coghill, Jeffrey G., and Christine Andresen. 2015. "Healthier U: Consumer Health for the Public." *Journal of Hospital Librarianship* 15:418–25. doi:10.1080/15323269.2015.1081011.

Couvillon, Emily, and Adela Justice. 2016. "Letters from the Big House: Providing Consumer Health Reference for Texas Prisons." *Journal of Hospital Librarianship* 16, no. 4: 281–86. http://dx/doi.org/10.1080/15323269.2016.1221272.

Davis, Jackie. 2013. "Health Information Ambassador Program for Patient Education: A Best Practice for Bringing the Consumer Health Library to the Patient." *Journal of Consumer Health on the Internet* 17, no. 1: 25–34. doi:10.1080/15398285.2013.756344.

Feeding America. 2017. "Child Hunger Fact Sheet." March 2017. http://www.feedingamerica.org/assets/pdfs/fact-sheets/child-hunger-fact-sheet.pdf.

Griggs, Judy. 2017. "Health Education Lesson Plan Kits: Fun and Useful for Community Health Education." *CAPHIS Consumer Connections* 33, no. 1 (January): n.p.

Henry County Library System. 2017. "Build a Better World: Building the Mind & Building the Body with Lunch at the Library!" http://www.henry.public.lib.ga.us/images/forms/HCLS-2017SFSP.pdf.

Mamo, Elizabeth, and Mary Ann Howie. 2017. "From the Library to the Bedside: Health Information Ambassador Program at Rochester General Hospital." *CAPHIS Consumer Connections* 33, no. 1 (January): n.p.

Marrapodi, Elisabeth. 2016. "Trinitas Regional Medical Center Library Consumer Outreach Project." *CAPHIS Consumer Connections* 32, no. 2 (June): 6.

McFadden, Laurie. 2017. "Berkeley College Collaborates with Local Public Library to Combat Hypertension." *CAPHIS Consumer Connections* 33, no. 3 (July): n.p.

Pima County Public Library. 2017. "Library Nurse." June 29, 2017. https://www.library pima.gov/public-health-nurse/.

Queens Library. n.d. "Summer Meals." http://www.queenslibrary.org/events/summer-meals.

Tuality Healthcare. 2016. *2016 Community Benefit Report*. https://www.tuality.org/tuality/themes/tuality/images/forms.THC_CommunityReport_2016.pdf.

Witman, Lydia. 2016. "New Patient & Family Library Service Wrapping Up Second Year." *CAPHIS Consumer Connections* 32, no. 3 (September): 5–8.

Index

Agency for Healthcare Research and Quality (AHRQ), "AHRQ Health Literacy Universal Precautions Toolkit," 3, 117–18; "Engage for Health: A Partnership for Improved Patient-Doctor Communications," partnership with NNLM/MAR, Pennsylvania Library Association, Hospital and Healthsystem Association of Pennsylvania, and NNLM/NEO, 103
Akron Children's Hospital, OH, "H.E.L.P." health education lesson plan kits for school, hospital, and community use, 139
Alternative Medicine, resources, 32–33
American Fact Finder (website), 4
American Indian Health (website), 116
American Library Association, 16; Core Values of Librarianship, 59, 100; Privacy Tool Kit, 66
Arctic Health (website), 116
AskMe3 (website), 29
Atchison County, MO, 16–17

Backman, Fredrick, xvii
Barnes, Susan J., 84–92
Baystate Health Consumer Health Library, MA, partnership with Chicopee Public Library, Logic Model, 87–88

Berkeley College School of Health Studies, NJ, partnership with Newark Public Library to host health fairs in honor of National High Blood Pressure Education Month, May 2017, 140
Brassil, Ellen, 87–88
BRCA testing, Angelia Jolie influence on, 130
Brower, Stewart, 15
Burroughs, Catherine M., 7, 83, 85

Cancer.gov (website), 27
CAPHIS (Consumer Health and Patient Information Section, MLA), 42
CDC (Centers for Disease Control and Prevention), "Plain Language Materials & Resources," 17
Census Bureau, US, 4
Channing Bete, fee-based consumer/patient materials, 44
Chicopee Public Library, partnership with Baystate Health Consumer Health Library, Logic Model, 87–88
Childhood Cancer Guides, 42
CINAHL (fee-based database), 41
ClinicalTrials.gov (website), 29
collection development policies, 35–39

145

Columbia County, NY, "Health Information on the Go: Reaching Rural Populations by Bookmobile," 51
Comics and Medicine Conference 2017, 44
Community Commons (website), 4
Community Health Status Indicators (CHIS) (website), 4
Community Hospital-Fairfax, MO, 16, 32–33
complementary medicine, resources, 32–33
Connecticut Consumer Health Information Network (Healthnet), ethical considerations providing reference services, 68
Connor, Elizabeth, 10
Consumer Health Complete (EBSCO Host fee-based database), 40–41
Consumer Health Specialization (MLA/NLM), 34, 59
Cooking for Good Health and Happiness, Laurel Public Library, DE, 51
Core Values of Librarianship (ALA), 59, 100
County Health Rankings & Roadmaps (website), 5
Cuban, Sondra, 6, 21

Davis, Jackie, 13, 92, 138
Dettmar, Nicole, 4, 7
Devine, Patricia J., 120
DIMRC, NLM's Disaster Information Management Research Center, 19–20
Disaster Information Specialization (NLM/MLA), 20
disclaimers, medical information, 24–26

East Brunswick Public Library, NJ, "Just for the Health of It," grant award from NNLM/MAR, 104
East Carolina University's Laupus Library, "Healthier U @ Your Library/Hospital," (course), 140
Easy Stats (website), 4
Engage for Health: A Partnership for Improved Patient-Doctor Communication, 103
EthnoMed (website), 115

Expecting the Best, ESL health and wellness curriculum, Center for Literacy Studies at the University of Tennessee, 106

Fairfax, MO, Community Hospital-Fairfax, 16
familydoctor.org (website), 27
FDA (Federal Drug Administration), mobile apps requirements, 124
Fenway Institute, 119
Finding Health Information Online, course taught by Judith Hayes, Tuality Healthcare Library, OR, 139
Florida Health Literacy Coalition, "Staying Healthy for Beginners," health literacy in ESL classes, 105
Focused Health Information Outreach program, NNLM/NER, 104
fotonovelas, 47
Foundation Center, 52
Frumento, Katherine Stemmer, 40

Gaiman, Neil, xviii
Gale Cengage Learning Health & Wellness Resource Center (fee-based database), 41
Gancarz, Anne, 87–88
Gay and Lesbian Medical Association, 119
Gay-Straight Alliance Network, 119–120
Genetics Home Reference (website), 29
Graphic Medicine (website), 44
Graphic Medicine Book Club Kits (NNLM/NER), 44–47
GREAT Customer Service Guidelines, University Library, University of Illinois at Urbana, 61
Greenwich Hospital, Medical Library Mission Statement, 40

Hackett, Martine, Ph.D., 63
Ham, Kelli, pushback from patron, 131
Hayes, Judith, Tuality Healthcare Library, OR, "Finding Health Information Online" course, 139
Health & Aging, NIH (website), 28
Health & Wellness Resource Center, (Gale Cengage fee-based database), 62

Health Awareness Through Library Outreach (HATLO), Suffolk Cooperative Library System NY, 140
healthfinder.gov (website), 27
Healthier U @ Your Library/Hospital, (course), 140
Health Information on the Go: Reaching Rural Populations by Bookmobile, Columbia County, NY, 51
Health Information Specialists Program, University of Oklahoma Health Sciences Center (OUHSC), 59–60
Health Information Translations (website), 115
HealthIT.gov, e-Health guidelines, 124–27
Health Literacy, component in ESL classes, 105–6; Helen Osborne, 106
"Health Literacy and Cultural Competence," NLM's National Information Center on Health Services Research and Care Technology (NICHSR) Health Services Research Information Council (HSRIC), 100
Healthnet: Connecticut Consumer Health Information Network, ethical considerations in providing reference services, 68
HealthReach (website), 116
Health sciences librarians, professional competencies (MLA), 59
H.E.L.P., Akron Children's Hospital, OH, health education plan kits for school, hospital, and community use, 139
Henry County Library System, GA, summer lunch program, 142
Hilton Publishing, fee-based consumer health materials, 42
Hmong Health Website, 116
Holt County, MO, 16–17
Household Products Database, 20
Howie, Mary Ann, 139
HSLANJ (Health Sciences Library Association of New Jersey), social media policy & guidelines, 128
Human Rights Campaign Healthcare Equity Index, 119

Illinois, University of at Urbana, University Library, GREAT Customer Service Guidelines, 61
iMedicalApps.com (website), 127
Indian Health Service, 17
Institute of Medicine, 3

Journeyworks, fee-based health promotion & educational materials, 44

Kaiser, Henry J. Family Foundation, 4
kidshealth.org (website), 30
Krames, fee-based consumer health materials, 44

Lab Tests Online (website), 41
Lake, Erica, xvii, 57, 59, 89
Laurel Public Library, DE, "Cooking for Good Health and Happiness," 51
Learning Health & Wellness Resource Center, (Gale Cengage fee-based database), 41
Leskovec, Jacqueline, 120
LibGuides, 24
Library Nurse, Pima County Public Library, Tucson, AZ, 141
LINCS, Library Information and Communication System, US Department of Education Office of Career, Technical, and Adult Education (OCTAE) research-based health literacy materials for ABE and ESL courses, 105–6
Louisiana State University, Shreveport Health Sciences Library, partnership with Shreve Memorial Library, healthy eating outreach for preschoolers, 51

Malachowski, Margot, 87–88
Mamo, Elizabeth, 139
Marcus, Cara, 11
Massachusetts Library System, 2, 8–9
McFadden, Laurie, 140
McKnight, Michelynn, 7
medical information disclaimers, 24–26
Medical Library Association, Disaster Information Specialization, 20;

Code of Ethics for Health Sciences Librarianship: Goals and Principles of Ethical Conduct, 100; Consumer Health Information Specialization, 34; Evaluate website guidelines, 26–27; Health Sciences Librarians Competencies, 59; MedlinePlus.gov (website), 28; "Top Ten Consumer Health Websites," 27–28
MedlinePlus Consumer Health Libraries, 10
MedlinePlus magazine, 43
Migration Policy Institute, 110
mission statements, 39–40
Mount Carmel Health Sciences Library, 7–8, 24; collection development policy, 35–36
Multicultural Health Information Resources, NNLM/MAR, Division of Specialized Information Services (SIS) (website), 116

Nassau County, NY, *Community Health Assessment 2014-2017*, 4–5, 15
National Institute on Aging's "Health & Aging," (website), 28
National Institutes of Health (NIH) Senior Health (website retired 2017), 28
NLM 4 Caregivers (website), 29
Noe, Michael, Graphic Medicine Specialist, NNLM/NER, 44–47
Nyugen, Tony, 120

Office of Refugee Resettlement, US, 5
Oklahoma, University of Health Sciences Center (OUHSC), Health Information Specialists Program, 59–60
Olney, Cynthia, 84–92
Orphanet (website), 29
Osborne, Helen, 106
Ottosen, Terri, "Prescription for Success: Consumer Health Information" course, 140

Pew Research Center, 1, 18, 21, 110, 123, 128
Physician Directories, online, 42–43
Pima County Public Library, AZ, Library Nurse, 141

Preston Medical Library, University of Tennessee Medical Center, Collection Development Policy, 36–38
Pricewaterhouse Cooper's Health Research Institute, 127
Prisons, Texas, consumer health information provided by Texas Medical Center, 141
"Professional Competencies for Health Sciences Librarians," MLA, 59
Promoting Health Literacy by Training Front-Line Staff in a Hospital Setting, Wilkes-Barre General Hospital, PA, 51
Prottsman, Mary Fran, 11
Providing Consumer Health Information to Patrons: A Workshop for Librarians, 60
PubMed (database), 41
PubMed Health (website), 29
Pushback from patron, Kelli Ham experience, 131

Queens (NY) Library, Mobile Health Information Classroom, 50; "English for Your Health," for ESL classes, 105; summer meal program, 142

Refugee Resettlement, US Office of, 5
Rochester General Hospital, NY, "Health Information Ambassador Program," 138–39
Roksandic, Stevo, Director, Mount Carmel Health System Library Services, 7, 24
Rural Health Information Hub (RHIhub), 4
Rural Women's Health Project (RWHP), fotonovelas, 47

Sackler, Richard and Jonathan Medical Library, Greenwich Hospital, CT, Mission Statement, 40
SAGE (Services & Advocacy for GLBT Elders), 119
Sandoval County, NM, 17
Shipman, Jean, xvii, 57, 59, 89
Shreve Memorial Library, LA, partnership with Louisiana State University's Shreveport Health Sciences Library,

health eating outreach to preschoolers, 51
SIS, Division of Specialized Information Services of NNLM/MAR, 116
Social media policy & guidelines, HSLANJ, 128
South Nassau Communities Hospital, "Community Service Plan, 2016–2018," 5; librarian participation in annual Health Fair/5K Run, 136; medical information disclaimer, 24–26
SPIRAL: Selected Patient Information Resources in Asian Languages (website), 116
Suffolk County, NY, *Community Health Assessment, 2014–2017*, 5, 16
summer lunch programs in libraries, 141–42

"Ten-Five" rule for customer service, 58
Tennessee, University of, Center for Literacy Studies, "Expecting the Best," ESL health and wellness curriculum, 106
Tennessee, University of, Medical Center Preston Medical Library, Collection Development Policy, 37–38
Texas Medical Center Library, consumer health information to inmates in 45 Texas prisons, 141
Tompkins-McCaw Library for the Health Sciences, Virginia Commonwealth Libraries, two-day workshop, "Providing Consumer Health Information to Patrons: A Workshop for Librarians," grant award from NNLM/SEA, 60
"Top Ten Consumer Health Websites," MLA, 27

ToxTown (website), 20
Trinitas Regional Medical Center, NJ, online health literacy site, 140
Tuality Healthcare Library, OR, community consumer health resource, and partnership with Washington County Cooperative Library System, 139

U.S. Census Bureau, 4
University of Oklahoma Health Sciences Center (OUHSC), Health Information Specialists Program, 59–60
University of Virginia, "Patient and Family Library," consumer health information service, 138
UpToDate (fee-based database), 40
Urban Indian Health Institute (UIHI), 85

Virginia Commonwealth Libraries, Tompkins-McCaw Library for the Health Sciences, two-day workshop, "Providing Consumer Health Information to Patrons: A Workshop for Librarians," grant award from NNLM/SEA, 60
Virginia, University of, "Patient and Family Library," consumer health information service, 138

WebMD, credibility, 33
Wikipedia, credibility of health-related topics, 129–30
WikiProject Med (WPMEF), 129
Wilkes-Barre General Hospital, PA, "Promoting Health Literacy by Training Front-Line Staff in Hospital Setting," 51
Witman, Lydia, 138
Wood, Fred B, 7, 83, 85

About the Author

Claire B. Joseph is director of the Medical Library at South Nassau Communities Hospital, Oceanside, Long Island, New York. She has been a librarian for more than forty years and a health sciences librarian for nearly thirty years. She is active in the Medical Library Association, serving as chair of the Hospital Libraries Section, chair-elect of the Nursing and Allied Health Resources Section, secretary of the Consumer and Patient Health Information Section, and chair of the New York-New Jersey Chapter, along with serving on a variety of committees. In addition, she is book review editor for the *Journal of Hospital Librarianship*.

www.ingramcontent.com/pod-product-compliance
Lightning Source LLC
Chambersburg PA
CBHW022014300426
44117CB00005B/183